Strengthen Your Mind Program

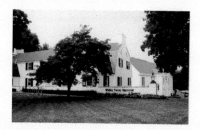

Also Available

Strengthen Your Mind

*Activities for People Concerned
About Early Memory Loss*

VOLUMES ONE AND TWO

By Kristin Einberger and Janelle Sellick, M.S.

Strengthen Your Mind Program

A Course for Memory Enhancement

by

Kristin Einberger

and

Janelle Sellick

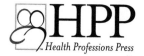
HPP
Health Professions Press

Baltimore • London • Sydney

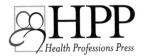

Health Professions Press, Inc.
Post Office Box 10624
Baltimore, Maryland 21285-0624

www.healthpropress.com

Typeset by Barton Matheson Willse & Worthington, Baltimore, Maryland.
Manufactured in the United States of America by Versa Press, East Peoria, Illinois.

Library of Congress Cataloging-in-Publication Data

Einberger, Kristin.
    Strengthen your mind program : a course for memory enhancement / by Kristin Einberger and Janelle Sellick.
        p. cm.
    Includes bibliographical references.
    ISBN 978-1-932529-55-5 (pbk.)
    1. Memory disorders in old age.   2. Memory disorders—Exercise therapy.   I. Sellick, Janelle.   II. Title.
    RC394.M46E354 2010
    616.85'230642—dc22
                                                                        2009040717

British Library Cataloguing in Publication data are available from the British Library.

Contents

Preface

One needs only to visit a bookstore to see how important memory improvement has become in recent years. Shelves are full of books on ways to strengthen the mind and maintain a sharp memory—eat foods rich in antioxidants, exercise more, learn a new language or instrument, engage all of the senses, socialize more. There are so many valuable techniques to learn and master and others to simply relearn and use more effectively. Healthy older adults, people concerned about their memory, and individuals diagnosed with an early memory loss disorder can all benefit from keeping their minds active.

We have been thrilled with the interest shown in volumes one and two of *Strengthen Your Mind: Activities for People Concerned About Early Memory Loss*, and continue to advocate for services for people with early memory loss. Through weekly early memory loss groups and presentations at various conferences throughout the United States, we have witnessed firsthand the need for resources designed specifically for people with early memory loss and those interested in enhancing their memory. We have also spoken with so many professionals (i.e., facilitators) who have expressed a desire to be able to teach a memory-improvement course, but who have not had the time or expertise to research, create, and plan such a course. To them, we offer this book. We hope that you enjoy teaching the 12 classes as much as we have enjoyed researching topics that are vital to memory as well as developing the tools and step-by-step approach to teach a course in memory enhancement.

As in the two previous volumes of *Strengthen Your Mind*, the practice activities in this book have been field-tested with individuals in our memory-enhancement classes to ensure that the topics are interesting and that the level of difficulty is appropriate. The groups with which we work continue to be our best teachers in designing and creating the content for this book. It is with much gratitude that we thank them!

Acknowledgments

We wish to dedicate this book to the hundreds of students to whom we have had the privilege of teaching memory enhancement techniques over the past few years. You have been our best teachers and for that we are eternally grateful.

From Kristin: I wish to thank my family and friends for their constant and endearing support of my writing efforts. They have all played an instrumental role in giving me the opportunity to do what I love. My special thanks go to my two sons, Derek and Scott, who have been and continue to be a huge inspiration in my work.

From Janelle: This book has been a joy to work on and I wouldn't have found it nearly as enjoyable if it weren't for the support and interest of my family. Thank you to my husband, Mike, for enduring my endless hours in front of the computer and for supporting and encouraging yet another writing endeavor. All my love to my three beautiful daughters, Megan, Mia, and Josie!

Introduction

This book is divided into 12 classes, each of which is meant to be taught in one session. Some topics, however, could lend themselves to multiple sessions, if desired. We have chosen 11 general topics that we believe are of significant importance to memory enhancement. The last class is a review of the previous 11 classes.

The amount of time to devote to each part of a class is given in parentheses and totals 90 minutes. These are suggested times only and should be adapted to meet the needs of the group and the facilitator. In larger groups especially, the class could easily last for 2 hours, as discussions may well be more lengthy. For each class, leave plenty of time for discussion, as this, in and of itself, is such an important component of enhancing one's memory.

For each class, the following information is included:

- An overview of the topic for the facilitator
- Step-by-step facilitator instructions
- A class agenda
- A warm-up activity, quiz, practice activities, handouts, and homework for class participants.

How to Use the Book

The facilitator should carefully review the overview before teaching a class to better understand the topic as well as any significant research related to the topic. The facilitator may then use the information throughout the class. Included in the facilitator overview are the following step-by-step instructions that explain how to teach the class.

Step One (Welcome and Introduction). The tasks that need to be done before class begins are listed first. Make all necessary copies of handouts for participants and pass them out as instructed. All handouts are listed in italics in both the facilitator instructions and the class agenda. Welcome the participants each day and let them know what the focus of that day's class will be. One or more quotes are included for each class. Writing them on a board or flip chart and then discussing their significance is a great way to set the tone for the class.

Step Two (Warm-Up Activity). The warm-up activity actively engages the participants. After giving everyone ample time to complete the activity, review the answers. In many cases an answer sheet is included for the facilitator.

Step Three (Quiz). The quiz, or in some cases a survey or questionnaire, is for all participants to complete. After everyone has had the chance to finish, review and discuss the responses or results.

Step Four (Explanation and Discussion). This is the heart of the class, and it is important to be very familiar with the overview before beginning this step. A thorough explanation of the topic should be given, using a board or flip chart, if possible, to optimize discussion and learning. Class discussion is very important. Attempt to gain feedback from as many participants as possible.

Step Five (Practice Activities). At this stage, participants are able to practice what has been taught. Using new information immediately is one of the best ways to retain the information, and this step allows participants the opportunity to do just that. The activities in this step are also designed to be enjoyable and interactive. Some of the activities may best be done individually, but doing them in groups of varying sizes is usually more advantageous.

Step Six (Review and Closing). For this step, it is important to give a quick overview of the class topic. Be sure to give participants the opportunity to ask questions. Thank the group for coming to class. It is also helpful to announce the topic of the next class in order to generate interest and enthusiasm.

Step Seven (Homework). When passing out the homework, explain what should be done for each assignment and remind participants of the value of completing the work. At least one homework assignment relates to the topic of the class and can, therefore, continue to strengthen the learning that has taken place. In some cases an answer sheet is included for the facilitator that may be handed out at the time the homework assignment is given or at the beginning of the next class. If the answer sheet is given at the time homework is passed out, it might be a good idea to fold it in half and staple it to discourage participants from checking the answers before they have completed the assignment. Remind participants that although completing the homework assignments individually is an excellent way to challenge their minds, for an added bonus they should try completing them with a friend or family member. Adding this social component makes for even broader mental stimulation (and is fun, too!).

Additional Information for Facilitators

The worksheets (warm-up activities, quizzes, practice activities, and homework assignments) are designed to be reproducible. We suggest making enough copies for each person in the group. You may also want to provide extra copies for people to take home with them so that they can work together on a topic with family members or friends. Make sure that participants are relaxed and focused on the topic before starting to work on an activity. When reviewing the questions, encourage people in the group to share their answers. Avoid just "reading off" the answers; take time to let people share any thoughts, memories, or stories that arise. Make the group feel comfortable by encouraging them to share or by sharing a story of your own. You can also ask them how they liked the worksheet, if they found it easy or difficult.

We suggest that you use a map for any worksheet that involves geography. For those that involve food, taste tests would be fun. For those that involve music, try bringing in different types of music and instruments and try encouraging singing. Using a variety of visual and auditory aids can be beneficial in working with any of the activities.

At the end of the book is a listing of resources that students in our memory-enhancement classes have found most helpful. If you have suggestions to add to future editions, feel free to e-mail us at keinberger81@gmail.com.

Although we have attempted to cover in this book many of the most significant topics related to memory enhancement, there are always more to be explored. Suggest to students that they explore some of these topics on their own.

Also, at the time of publication we attempted to cover some of the latest research. In our fast-moving, ever-changing society, new discoveries and research are constantly announced. Facilitators may want to check the Internet for the most up-to-date information on any of the 11 topics prior to teaching each individual class.

Memory and Aging

Memory and Aging
FACILITATOR OVERVIEW

We are lucky to be living in a time when so much research and interest in mental fitness is taking place. Over the past 10 to 15 years researchers have made huge advances in their knowledge of how the brain works, and how we can keep it sharp as we age. For the topic of memory and aging, participants will discuss myths about the aging brain and learn about important concepts related to memory, such as brain plasticity and neurogenesis. In addition, participants will learn about the three types of memory as well as what changes in the brain are to be expected as a person ages.

Your brain is a fascinating organ capable of feats that continue to amaze researchers and citizens alike. This overview is just the beginning of many important and fun facts about the brain—all of which will come to light in the classes that follow.

NORMAL AGE-RELATED CHANGES IN MEMORY

Contrary to what many people believe, memory loss is not an inevitable part of aging. In fact, there are many people who live into their 80s, 90s, and beyond who have a memory that is "sharp as a tack." There are some changes in memory, however, that are to be expected, including the following:

- *It takes longer to process new information.* It is more difficult to learn a new skill or to read and understand a lengthy magazine article.

- *It takes longer to recall information.* Whereas you may have been able to recall events, names, and facts quickly in the past, it may take longer to recall information (i.e., "tip of the tongue syndrome," wherein you know the answer but just cannot quite pull the information from your memory).

- *It becomes more difficult to pay attention to more than one thing at a time.* As a person ages, multitasking becomes more and more challenging. In fact, it can be said that multitasking is the enemy of memory. In the past you may have been able to cook dinner, talk on the phone, and feed the dog, but you may now find doing all three tasks at once an experience that leaves you frustrated.

Why does it become more difficult to multitask? One study reported by O'Brien (2008) suggests that the brain loses its capacity to ignore irrelevant information as a person grows older. In the study, participants had difficulty suppressing unnecessary information, which directly correlated to how well they did on a memory test.

Although most of the aging population worries about memory, for most people memory complaints are minimal and do not interfere with daily life. If you are truly concerned, try keeping a record of things that you forget and asking a family member or a close friend if he or she has noticed lapses in your memory. Finally, speak with your doctor about your concerns and consider an appointment for a full neurological workup to diagnose or dismiss a form of dementia, such as Alzheimer's disease.

When is memory loss cause for concern? Although it is difficult to tell, some warning signs include:

- Repeating stories or questions more than usual

- Difficulty performing routine tasks (loading the dishwasher)

- Problems with abstract thinking or numbers (balancing the checkbook)

- Forgetting conversations or an appointment

- Misplacing items or putting them in strange locations (sugar bowl in the refrigerator)

- Becoming easily distracted or disoriented

- Changes in personality, such as mood swings, lack of trust in others, depression, isolation, or anxiety.

Although these symptoms can be concerning, for most people changes in memory are a part of normal aging. While some changes, such as "tip of the tongue syndrome," may cause frustration, the brain is capable of other changes that can actually help to improve memory.

BRAIN PLASTICITY

According to Finnemore (2009), neuroplasticity (or brain plasticity) is the brain's capacity to learn and remember new information in response to influences and experiences as a person ages. What does this mean for memory? It means that the brain is more than able to learn new information, create new ideas, and, most important, change in response to learning. According to Nelson (2005), a person continues to grow new neurons, or nerve cells, throughout life, a process called *neurogenesis*. This ability to grow new nerve cells is what allows and supports brain plasticity. Although it is true that we lose thousands of brain cells each day, new ones can be created. In fact, in normal aging there is no significant loss of nerve cells in key areas of the brain's hippocampus, which is the most important structure for memory (Nelson, 2005).

Whereas it used to be thought that "you can't teach an old dog new tricks," we now know that even as people grow older they are able to learn and challenge their brains. Some studies even suggest that people with early Alzheimer's disease can still learn new information. Two studies supported by the National Institute on Aging found that mildly impaired participants with Alzheimer's disease improved their ability to recall faces as well as to respond to and process information more rapidly. In addition, the study participants, who received 3 to 4 months of cognitive therapy, were better oriented to time and place as compared to another group of patients with Alzheimer's disease who did not receive cognitive therapy.

TYPES OF MEMORY

Some of the most common complaints regarding memory loss and aging concern short-term memory. People often report losing their keys, forgetting why they came into a room, or having trouble remembering names. There are actually three types of memory, each of which plays an important role in a person's ability to remember.

Sensory Memory

Any information that the brain processes first passes through sensory memory. In fact, we are bombarded with more stimuli than we even realize because sensory memory acts as a filter, deciding which information is important enough to hold on to. Sensory memory is extremely short, lasting only milliseconds. Because we receive so many stimuli, each sensory experience erases the last. That is, if sensory memory deems a stimulus important, it is immediately passed on to short-term memory.

Short-term Memory

According to Nelson (2005), short-term memory is information that you need to remember for just a few seconds or minutes. For example, your short-term memory is at work if you try to remember a phone number just long enough to dial it. After you take action, it is gone. The amount of information that your short-term memory can hold is about five to nine items, with seven being the average. That is why we find it easier to remember a phone number or social security number than a longer number, such as for a bank account. Similar to sensory memory, short-term memory acts as a filter to keep information that is not important from cluttering up long-term memory. Without short-term memory, the brain would be full of useless facts, ideas, and numbers, which would make it extremely difficult to go about daily life.

Long-term Memory

Long-term memory is the virtually limitless information that has been gathered throughout a person's life. According to Higbee (1996), short-term memory is like an inbox on a desk, whereas long-term memory is like a large file cabinet. Something that is personally important or striking will likely be transferred to long-term memory. Most people can remember details about their wedding day, their first car, or what they did for their first job. Other events, with broader social or historical significance, are also easily stored in long-term memory. For example, most people can recall where they were when John F. Kennedy was assassinated or what they were doing on September 11, 2001. In addition, long-term memory stores much of the information that we rely on in daily life, to be retrieved when needed—how to brush our teeth, which route to drive to work, social etiquette and manners.

Memory and Aging
FACILITATOR INSTRUCTIONS

1. WELCOME AND INTRODUCTION (10 MINUTES)

To do before class:

- Read and familiarize yourself with the Memory and Aging Overview.

- Write the following quotes on a board or flip chart.

> "Every man's memory is his private literature."
> (Aldous Huxley, author)

> "Memory is a child walking along a seashore. You can never tell what small pebble it will pick up and store away among its treasured things."
> (Pierce Harris, columnist, *Atlanta Journal*)

- Familiarize yourself with and make appropriate copies of the warm-up activity, quiz, practice activities, and homework.

Greet the class and have the participants introduce themselves, if necessary. Explain that the purpose of the class is to dispel some of the myths about memory and to learn about some of the important processes related to keeping memory sharp as you age. Tell the participants that they will be working on plenty of practice activities to get their brains warmed up and ready for the next 11 weeks of memory enhancement classes!

Discuss the quotes and ask participants for their interpretations. Ask the class how memory shapes us as individuals. Do participants experience times when their memory fails them? How about when their memory surprises them?

2. WARM-UP ACTIVITY (10 MINUTES)

Distribute the worksheet *Creating Words* and explain that this activity is a way to get participants' brains warmed up for the class ahead. In addition, this exercise is an excellent brain booster, because it forces participants to "think outside the box." After about 5 minutes, give each person a chance to share some of his or her answers.

3. MEMORY QUIZ (15 MINUTES)

There are many myths about the aging brain and what happens to memory as a person grows older. Pass out the *Memory Quiz* and explain that it will address some of these "gray areas" and attempt to clear up any uncertainty about memory loss and aging. Tell participants just to do the best they can. If they do not know an answer, they are welcome to leave it blank. After about 5 minutes or when it looks as though most have finished, go over the answers to the quiz and pause for questions and comments.

4. EXPLANATION AND DISCUSSION OF MEMORY AND AGING OVERVIEW (15 MINUTES)

Explain to participants that although memory loss is *not* a normal part of aging, there are three common age-related changes in memory that participants can expect. Explain the three bulleted changes in the overview. Ask participants if they have experienced any of the changes and how it felt. Has anyone come up with a way to handle "tip of the tongue syndrome" or the frustrations that come with multitasking? Explain that although most people will not experience significant memory loss, some signs of memory loss could be serious. Read the bulleted list of warning signs and explain that it is always best to speak with a doctor or loved one if a participant is truly concerned about his or her memory.

Explain that the good news about the aging brain is that no matter how old you are you can still challenge your brain and learn new information. Review the section on brain plasticity and emphasize that people can make their brains stronger by exercising them, just like they exercise their bodies.

Finally, review the section on the three types of memory and explain the importance of each one. Most problems with memory occur with short-term memory (e.g., losing keys or forgetting a person's name, appointments, or why you walked into a room). Explain that in this class participants will learn tricks for remembering as well as tips for how to improve memory in general.

5. PRACTICE ACTIVITIES (30 MINUTES)

Before beginning the group activity, Experiencing Your Sensory Memory, refer the class back to the three types of memory and emphasize that sensory memory is so good at filtering out unnecessary information that we often do not even realize what sounds, sights, and other stimuli are all around us. Ask participants to close their eyes for one minute and take note of the sounds and smells around them. Then ask participants to open their eyes and take a minute to really look around the room. What things did they hear, smell, or see that they would not have noticed before? Thank goodness for sensory memory for filtering out most of these things that are not necessary for us to be aware of all at once!

Pass out the worksheet *I'm Good at Remembering*. Explain to the class that most people have a tendency to focus on the negative things about their memory ("I can never remember names!"). For this exercise participants will try to list at least five things that they are good at remembering. After each person has filled out the worksheet, ask for volunteers to share what they have written. Explain that negative thoughts about memory can become a self-fulfilling prophecy (the group will learn more about this as part of the class on Optimism and Humor), and that focusing on what they can remember will help to reframe the way they think about memory.

6.   REVIEW AND CLOSING (5 MINUTES)

Thank everyone for their participation in the class and ask if anyone has any final questions. Explain that in the next 11 classes participants will learn about all aspects of memory and how to improve it. Review the main concepts introduced in this class and encourage participants to challenge their brains on a regular basis.

7.   HOMEWORK (5 MINUTES)

Pass out the homework sheets, explain what should be done for each, and encourage everyone to complete them during the week. Explain that the homework is for fun, but that it also helps to challenge the brain and make it stronger. As participants do each homework sheet they are actually growing new brain cells!

- *Animal Names Spelled with Three and Four Letters*

- *Ways to Challenge Your Brain A–Z*

- Try to incorporate into your life this week at least one or two new ideas from your Ways to Challenge Your Brain A–Z list.

Memory and Aging
CLASS AGENDA

1. Welcome and Introduction
2. Warm-Up Activity
   - *Creating Words*
3. Memory Quiz
4. Overview of Memory and How It Changes as We Age
   - Normal Age-Related Changes in Memory
   - Brain Plasticity
   - Types of Memory
5. Practice Activities
   - Experiencing Your Sensory Memory (Group Activity)
   - *I'm Good at Remembering . . .*
6. Review and Closing
7. Homework
   - *Animal Names Spelled with Three and Four Letters*
   - *Ways to Challenge Your Brain A–Z*
   - Try to incorporate at least one or two new ideas from *Ways to Challenge Your Brain A–Z* into your life this week!

Strengthen Your Mind Program: A Course for Memory Enhancement by Einberger & Sellick.

Creating Words

Challenge your brain with this warm-up activity. Think of a word or words for each category that begins with each letter of the word *brain*.

Categories	B	R	A	I	N
Places					
Items in your kitchen					
Animals					
Famous people					

Memory Quiz

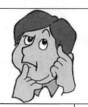

Write *T* for *true* or *F* for *false* on the line before each statement.

_____   1.   The majority of older people (age 65 or older) are senile.

_____   2.   Advancing age can cause memory loss.

_____   3.   Depression can affect memory.

_____   4.   Once brain cells are lost, more cannot be created.

_____   5.   *Short-term memory* refers to something that has happened in the last month.

_____   6.   It can take older people longer than younger people to recall information.

_____   7.   Poor nutrition can cause memory loss.

_____   8.   Problems with memory can often be attributed to lack of ˙focus.

_____   9.   Age in itself does little to affect a person's ability to learn.

_____   10.   Your short-term memory is the first stop for information coming into your brain.

Strengthen Your Mind Program: A Course for Memory Enhancement by Einberger & Sellick.

Memory Quiz ANSWER SHEET

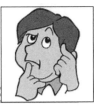

__F__ 1. **The majority of older people (age 65 or older) are senile.**
Only about 5% of people over age 65 have some form of dementia. The word *senile* is actually an out-of-date medical term that was used to differentiate age of onset of dementia. The term *dementia* is used today instead of *senile*. It is important, however, to remember that dementia itself is not a diagnosis; a disease or other problem is always the cause of dementia.

__F__ 2. **Advancing age can cause memory loss.**
Growing older does not cause memory loss. Certain changes in memory can be expected as a person ages (we will go over these changes in class today); however, losing memory is not one of them.

__T__ 3. **Depression can affect memory.**
Mild depression can cause problems with memory, and depression can mimic symptoms of dementia. If depression is diagnosed and treatment is started, improvements in memory often occur.

__F__ 4. **Once brain cells are lost, more cannot be created.**
New brain cells can be created at any age.

__F__ 5. ***Short-term memory* refers to something that has happened in the last month.**
Short-term memory refers to something that has happened in the last few seconds or minutes.

__T__ 6. **It can take older people longer than younger people to recall information.**
As you age it does take longer to recall information; however, even though it may take longer to recall, in normal aging the information always does eventually come to you.

__T__ 7. **Poor nutrition can cause memory loss.**
Lack of B vitamins in your diet, specifically vitamins B_6 and B_{12}, can cause memory loss that can mimic symptoms of dementia.

__T__ 8. **Problems with memory can often be attributed to lack of focus.**
Not focusing on what you are doing is an enemy of memory. In order to remember something, you must really pay attention and focus 100%.

__T__ 9. **Age in itself does little to affect a person's ability to learn.**
We are able to learn new information at any age.

__F__ 10. **Your short-term memory is the first stop for information coming into your brain.**
Information coming into your brain first passes through your sensory memory, then on to your short-term memory.

Strengthen Your Mind Program: A Course for Memory Enhancement by Einberger & Sellick.
© 2010 by Health Professions Press, Inc.

I'm Good at Remembering . . .

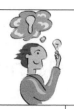

Many people focus on the things they cannot remember more than the things they can. Think about the things that you are good at remembering and list at least five. *Thinking positively about your memory can help you to remember!*

1.

2.

3.

4.

5.

Strengthen Your Mind Program: A Course for Memory Enhancement by Einberger & Sellick.

Animal Names Spelled with Three and Four Letters

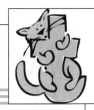

Name 12 animals that are spelled with three letters.

1.   7.

2.   8.

3.   9.

4.   10.

5.   11.

6.   12.

Name 12 animals that are spelled with four letters.

1.   7.

2.   8.

3.   9.

4.   10.

5.   11.

6.   12.

Ways to Challenge Your Brain A–Z

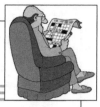

There are many ways of "exercising" your brain. One of the most common is to do crossword puzzles. Challenge your brain right now by thinking of a brain exercise that begins with each letter of the alphabet. Be creative!

A

B

C

D

E

F

G

H

I

J

K

L

M

N

O

P

Q

R

S

T

U

V

W

X

Y

Z

Strengthen Your Mind Program: A Course for Memory Enhancement by Einberger & Sellick.

Learning Styles

Learning Styles
FACILITATOR OVERVIEW

Learning styles are different ways in which a person processes information in order to learn it and apply it. We all learn in different ways. Some of us learn best by seeing, others by listening, and still others by doing. Whether we can actually learn depends in large part on whether the information is presented in a way consistent with our primary learning style. For people who are auditory learners, hearing and processing new information out loud works best. Visual learners need to be able to see things, to read things, and to take notes. Those who are tactile/kinesthetic learners need to touch and feel things and prefer hands-on learning.

It is important for all of us to remember that each of us is unique in how we learn best. It is easy to assume that because someone may learn best by reading instructions before starting to assemble something that others learn best in the same way. Others may prefer to use an auditory or tactile/kinesthetic style to learn. For this reason, and as this lesson will teach, it is particularly important to use all three learning styles when teaching and explaining information to be learned so as to engage each participant's learning style. Whereas in the past instruction was mainly given in lecture form, focusing primarily on the auditory learning style, over the past few decades we have come to realize that in order for students to remember best, be they age 8 or 80, instruction should incorporate all three learning styles. For example, if a lesson focuses on learning how to use the Internet, students not only need to hear how to use it, but also to see examples of how it is used and to have hands-on experience using it.

Below is a summary of the characteristics of each learning style:

Visual Learners

• Learn best by being able to see things, including facial expressions and body language

• Are distracted by visual stimuli and movement around them

• Need to see things in written form rather than just hear information about them

• Dislike listening for too long

Auditory Learners

• Learn best by hearing things

• Are easily distracted by noise

• Are sensitive to how things sound in the environment

• Often have trouble with written directions when they are not accompanied by oral ones

Tactile/Kinesthetic Learners

- Need to be able to touch and feel things and prefer hands-on learning

- Have difficulty sitting still for too long and need to be able to move around

- Are distracted by things going on around them in which they are not involved

- Learn better when physical activity is involved

Handouts are included for each learning style that describe in more depth the characteristics of each and specific ways to focus on using an individual learning style. It is extremely important when teaching all of the lessons in this book to include techniques that are appropriate for each learning style, not just the one that you, the facilitator, learn best by. Besides lecturing, use visual aids such as maps, charts, and graphs. Also, use hands-on materials that the participants can actually touch (props, highlighters, and things to pass around, such as books and pictures).

In this lesson, participants will gain a greater understanding of which learning style is dominant for them. At the same time, however, they will come to appreciate that learning to use the other learning styles more effectively increases the chances of remembering what they learn.

Learning Styles
FACILITATOR INSTRUCTIONS

1. WELCOME AND INTRODUCTION (10 MINUTES)

To do before class:

- Read and familiarize yourself with the Learning Styles Overview.

- Review the characteristics and tips for each style of learning.

- Write the following quotes on a board or flip chart.

> You don't understand anything until you learn it more than one way.
> (Marvin Minsky, scientist)

> We learn by example and by direct experience because there are real
> limits to the adequacy of verbal instruction.
> (Malcolm Gladwell, author)

- Set out 8–10 items as described in the warm-up activity. Cover them so that participants cannot see them before the activity begins.

- Familiarize yourself with and make appropriate copies of the quiz, practice activities, and homework.

Welcome the participants and let them know that the focus of the class will be learning styles and how we can use each one to enhance memory. Explain that individuals learn in different ways—some by seeing, some by hearing, and some by doing. Ask participants if they believe they learn best by seeing things, by hearing things, or by touching things. Explain that everyone will have the opportunity to explore the way or ways by which they learn best.

Discuss the quotes and ask participants for their interpretations. What does Mr. Minsky mean in saying that you have to learn something in more than one way? How do we do this? In the Gladwell quote, is verbal instruction really not enough for most of us?

2. WARM-UP ACTIVITY (10 MINUTES)

Uncover the 8–10 items you have set out on a table in the middle of the room. Some of the items should have an associated sound. Items may include:

- a baby rattle

- chalk

- a musical instrument

- a photo
- a certificate
- a can
- a map
- a piece of fruit
- a stapler
- a pen
- a calculator
- a dollar bill

Give participants 2 minutes to study the items in whichever way they like. Take the items away and ask them to name as many of the items as they can. How did they remember each item? Did they make a list (visual); did they say the names of the items out loud (auditory); did they touch the items (tactile/kinesthetic)? Which technique(s) (learning style) worked best?

3. LEARNING STYLES QUIZ (10 MINUTES)

Give participants ample time to complete the 15 questions for the quiz *Which Learning Style Are You?* After completion, ask participants to score their quiz, counting how many As, Bs, and Cs they circled. Tell them that the As are for visual learners, the Bs for auditory learners, and the Cs for tactile/kinesthetic learners. In which learning style did they score the highest? The lowest? Let everyone know that they will be able to use this information to learn memory skills that are especially appropriate for them.

4. EXPLANATION AND DISCUSSION OF LEARNING STYLES AND HOW THEY AFFECT MEMORY (30 MINUTES)

List the three learning styles on a board or flip chart. Explain to participants that each of us learns in different ways and that this class will help each of them determine which learning style they use most frequently as well as the characteristics of that learning style. They will also learn tips for using each learning style that will allow them to strengthen their preferred style as well as increase the use of their nondominant styles.

Distribute the three learning styles handouts and review each one by one, first discussing the characteristics and then the tips for using each style. Ask participants to share any other tips they have found useful. Discuss how easily these tips can be practiced to improve memory.

5. PRACTICE ACTIVITIES (20 MINUTES)

There are many ways to practice using the different learning styles. Try one on remembering names. Pick a name, such as George. Distribute the handout *Remembering a Person's Name Using Each Learning Style.* Ask participants for suggestions on how to remember the name George using each learning style. Give them 3–4 minutes to develop their own list.

- Visual learning style examples:

1. Write the name repeatedly.

2. Think of a "picture" of someone else with the name, such as George W. Bush or Curious George.

•   Auditory learning style examples:

1. Repeat the name a few times out loud.

2. Use the name as many times as possible in conversation with the person, such as "Nice to meet you, George" or "I hope to see you again, George." Always say the name out loud.

•   Tactile/Kinesthetic learning style examples:

1. "Write" the name in the air a few times.

2. Use a motor cue associated with the name, such as chopping down a tree for George Washington.

Review participant responses.

Another practice activity could be remembering a short grocery list. Ask for suggestions on how to remember the list using each of the three learning styles (e.g., write out the list a few times, say it out loud, imagine how each item would feel).

Yet another activity could be to divide the participants into 2–3 groups and give each group one of the following brainstorming tasks:

•   You are putting together a menu for a big party. How would you use each learning style in making preparations?

•   You are assembling a bicycle for your child's birthday gift. How would you use each learning style to put it together?

•   A group of friends is helping you organize your kitchen. How would you use each learning style to assure that everyone can take part in this chore?

6.   REVIEW AND CLOSING (5 MINUTES)

Thank the group for their participation. Review the main characteristics of the three learning styles and a couple of tips for each. Remind participants that although we tend to use our dominant learning style most frequently, it is also important to use *all* three when learning new information or reviewing that which has already been learned. Most of us learn best in one way, but as Marvin Minsky stated (point out the quote on the board), it is important to learn something in more than one way to really understand it best.

7.   HOMEWORK (5 MINUTES)

Pass out the homework sheets and review what should be done for each. Remind participants that it is important that they use what they have learned in class to complete the homework and try to incorporate ways to use each of the learning styles in their daily lives. Also remind them of the importance of completing homework assignments in order to best remember what they have learned!

•   *An Imaginary Trip to Italy*

•   *Words that Rhyme* (possible answers are included)

•   Have participants review how they learn best and study the tips for that learning style, using as many of the tips as possible.

Learning Styles
CLASS AGENDA

1. Welcome and Introduction
2. Warm-Up Activity
   - Study the Items! (Group Activity)
3. Learning Styles Quiz—*Which Learning Style Are You?*
4. Overview of Learning Styles and Tips for Each Type of Learner
   - *Visual Learners*
   - *Auditory Learners*
   - *Tactile/Kinesthetic Learners*
5. Practice Activities
   - *Remembering a Name Using Each Learning Style*
   - How to Remember a Short Grocery List (Group Activity)
   - Brainstorming (Group Activity)
6. Review and Closing
7. Homework
   - *An Imaginary Trip to Italy*
   - *Words that Rhyme*
   - Practice using *all* three learning styles in your daily life!

Which Learning Style Are You?

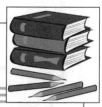

By answering the following questions, you will gain a basic idea of which learning style you use most often. For a more in-depth assessment, you can find a number of quizzes on the Internet.

1. **When I talk with my friends on the phone . . .**

    A. It's difficult to listen for too long because I can't see them.

    B. I enjoy both listening and talking.

    C. I gesture often and nod my head, even though they can't see me.

2. **When I want to relax, I'm more likely to . . .**

    A. Watch a movie or visit a local exhibit.

    B. Listen to special music or have a conversation with a friend.

    C. Do something active where I can use my hands.

3. **At a sporting event . . .**

    A. I love to watch all that's going on.

    B. It's important for me to listen to the announcer.

    C. I often wish I were involved in the activity myself.

4. **When I need to go somewhere I haven't been before, I'm more likely to . . .**

    A. Look at a map and write out directions for myself.

    B. Ask someone for verbal directions.

    C. Go with my gut instinct of where it is.

5. **When I'm putting together a new shelf . . .**

    A. I read the directions first and appreciate pictures and diagrams.

    B. I read directions aloud or have them read to me.

    C. I don't necessarily look at the directions—I just jump right in.

    D. I hire someone else to get it done. (Just kidding—this doesn't count!)

6. **When choosing a new book to read, I'm more likely to . . .**

    A. Choose one with vivid descriptions and/or pictures so that I can *see* what's going on.

    B. Choose one with a lot of conversation so that I can *hear* what's going on.

    C. Choose one with a lot of action so that I can actually *feel* what's going on.

Strengthen Your Mind Program: A Course for Memory Enhancement by Einberger & Sellick.

7. **When I really want to concentrate on something . . .**

    A. I'm distracted by clutter and movement around me.

    B. I'm distracted by sounds/noise in the area.

    C. I'm distracted when there's a lot going on around me.

8. **When I buy new clothes . . .**

    A. I pick them primarily for how they look.

    B. I pay special attention to sounds they make, such as the swishing of silk.

    C. I pick them for how they feel.

9. **When I watch a musical on television or at the movies, I am more likely to . . .**

    A. Concentrate on what's most visually appealing to me.

    B. Concentrate on the sounds/songs I like best.

    C. Pay special attention to how the music and dialogue make me feel.

10. **The best way for me to remember an object is to . . .**

    A. Picture it in my head and study how it looks.

    B. Imagine the sounds it makes.

    C. Pick it up and study how it feels.

11. **When working in a group, I need to . . .**

    A. See everyone's facial expressions and watch their body language.

    B. Listen carefully and talk things through with others.

    C. Move, do, touch, and be hands on.

12. **When trying to remember a few items I need at the grocery store and I'm unable to make a list, I . . .**

    A. Visualize the items in my head and think about where they are in the store.

    B. Repeat the list out loud a few times and/or have someone repeat it to me.

    C. Visualize the feel of the items and imagine myself walking through the store to find them.

13. **When listening to a lecture . . .**

    A. I watch the presenter and like to take notes about the content.

    B. I listen carefully and may even record the lecture in order to be able to listen to it again later.

    C. I often doodle, move frequently in my seat, or stand to listen.

14. If another person were to ask me if I understood something they were saying, I would likely say something like . . .

    A. That looks right.

    B. That sounds right.

    C. That feels right.

15. I remember best by

    A. Seeing.

    B. Hearing.

    C. Doing.

SCORING

Number of As _____

Number of Bs _____

Number of Cs _____

As focus on the visual learning style
Bs focus on the auditory learning style
Cs focus on the tactile/kinesthetic learning style

Your highest number is the dominant learning style you use to process information.

Strengthen Your Mind Program: A Course for Memory Enhancement by Einberger & Sellick.

Visual Learners

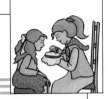

CHARACTERISTICS

- Need to *see* something to know it.
- Need to see body language and facial expressions.
- Have a strong sense of color.
- May have artistic ability.
- Have difficulty with *spoken* directions.
- Are distracted by movement or untidiness. Like things to be neat and in order. Appearance is very important.
- Tend to be relatively unaware of noise.
- Prefer to sit in the front of a room for a meeting, lecture, discussion, etc.
- Dislike listening for too long.
- Need to see something in written form rather than just hear about it.
- Forget names but remember faces.
- Use visual-type phrases, such as "I see," "Just imagine," or "I've never looked at it that way before."

TIPS FOR VISUAL LEARNERS

- Stand in front of people when listening or interacting.
- Challenge yourself regularly with visual games and puzzles.
- Illustrate your ideas as a picture or diagram when you want to remember something.
- Use multimedia, such as videos, computers, etc.
- Read illustrated books. When using a cookbook, it's better to use one with pictures. When assembling an item, the directions, both written and illustrated, are very important.
- Visualize information or compose mental pictures as a memorization aid.
- Use color-coded systems to organize notes, cabinets, etc. Using highlighters with written information can be particularly helpful.
- Write out lists, notes, and reminders.
- Use a calendar.
- Minimize visual distractions, including glare in a room.
- Work in a well-lit area whenever possible.
- Watch the body language of the person to whom you are speaking.

Auditory Learners

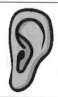

CHARACTERISTICS

- Prefer to learn information by *listening*.
- Have difficulty following written directions.
- Easily distracted by noise or extraneous activity.
- More likely to absorb reading material when read out loud.
- Enjoy lectures and discussions with other people.
- Hearing loss is especially problematic for an auditory learner, because it can lead to isolation and depression.
- May forget faces, but will often remember names.
- Need to talk things out.
- Sensitive to how things sound in the environment.
- Use auditory-type phrases, such as "I hear you" or "That doesn't sound right to me."

TIPS FOR AUDITORY LEARNERS

- Give yourself time to respond to verbal questions and cues.
- Eliminate as much background noise as possible.
- Don't shout when you think someone doesn't hear you, and ask those with whom you are speaking not to shout at you, but rather to speak in a normal voice.
- Sit near the person who is speaking.
- Ask those with whom you are speaking not to chew gum or put their hands over their mouth, because this makes it more difficult (or impossible) to understand what they are saying.
- Repeat or rehearse new information, names, or facts out loud.
- Make up rhymes to remember things, such as "*i* before *e* except after *c*."
- Participate in group discussions, and don't be afraid to ask questions or ask someone to repeat what he or she said.
- Read out loud.
- Discuss your ideas verbally.
- Use a tape recorder to hear information again.
- Teach new information to someone else soon after you learn it.

Strengthen Your Mind Program: A Course for Memory Enhancement by Einberger & Sellick.

Tactile/Kinesthetic Learners

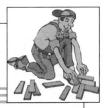

CHARACTERISTICS

- Prefer *hands-on* learning and projects.
- Can often assemble parts without reading directions.
- Have difficulty sitting still. Like to move around.
- Are distracted by activity in which they're not involved.
- Learn better when physical activity is involved.
- May be very well coordinated.
- React well to group work.
- Use gestures.
- Doodle while learning.
- Have the most trouble in settings in which they are expected to sit down and listen in a solitary way, such as in a classroom or lecture.
- Use tactile/kinesthetic-type phrases, such as "I feel" or "That doesn't feel right" or "That really touched me."

TIPS FOR TACTILE/KINSTHETIC LEARNERS

- Increase movement. Move around to learn new things.
- Move and stretch between or during activities.
- Take frequent breaks.
- Use all senses as much as possible.
- Feel, touch, and smell items as much as possible.
- Write out facts several times in order to learn them.
- Participate actively (construct, draw, "show and tell").
- Work in a standing position when appropriate.
- Develop "motor cues" to learn names, such as swinging a bat to remember someone's name who really likes baseball.
- Take opportunities to work on crossword puzzles and to play Scrabble, card games, and a variety of other mentally stimulating activities, all of which are good exercises for improving memory and involve touching things.
- Highlight items that you want to remember. Don't be afraid to doodle.
- Use flashcards while learning new information, such as the seven continents or important numbers you need to remember.

Remembering a Person's Name Using Each Learning Style

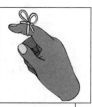

Write the name of a person on the line below and describe how you could learn to remember it using each of the three learning styles.

NAME _____

Using the visual learning style:

Using the auditory learning style:

Using the tactile/kinesthetic learning style:

Strengthen Your Mind Program: A Course for Memory Enhancement by Einberger & Sellick.
© 2010 by Health Professions Press, Inc.

An Imaginary Trip to Italy

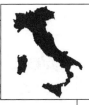

Imagine taking a vacation to Italy. How could you prepare for your trip using each of the three learning styles?

Using the visual learning style:

Using the auditory learning style:

Using the tactile/kinesthetic learning style:

Words that Rhyme

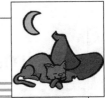

Name at least one word that rhymes with each of the following. Use your imagination.

bed

rock

paper

cup

jingle

pen

busted

turn

chide

dotted

drab

quick

board

flying

green

skated

mind

tools

styles

handle

zoo

Strengthen Your Mind Program: A Course for Memory Enhancement by Einberger & Sellick.

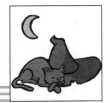

Words that Rhyme ANSWER SHEET

bed
red, dead, wed, fed, head, led, lead

rock
sock, stock, jock, balk, chalk, walk, talk, mock, knock, lock

paper
caper, draper, taper

cup
pup, sup

jingle
shingle, mingle, single

pen
den, when, yen, ten, wren, men, hen

busted
rusted, trusted, lusted

turn
burn, churn, fern, learn

chide
bide, tide, side, wide, guide, hide

dotted
spotted, slotted, rotted, knotted

drab
cab, gab, jab, lab, nab, tab

quick
pick, stick, wick, tick, sick, kick, lick, knick, hick, chick, slick

board
bored, stored, ignored, cord, ford, gourd, hoard, lord

flying
buying, tying, sighing, dying

green
seen, bean, dean, lean, mean, preen, wean, teen

skated
baited, waited, mated, hated, dated

mind
kind, bind, blind, wind, signed, rind, find, hind, dined, lined

tools
rules, cools, drools, fools

styles
riles, dials, guiles, miles, tiles, whiles

handle
candle, scandal

zoo
boo, coo, do, lieu, moo, new, too, sue, woo, you

Mental Aerobics

Mental Aerobics
FACILITATOR OVERVIEW

It is widely known that exercising your brain is important as you get older. Memory clubs, computer games, and trivia books are becoming mainstream as the aging population recognizes that people can do something about memory loss and work to keep their memory sharp as they age. Crossword puzzles are one of the most popular mental-aerobic activities. There are, however, many, many other fun activities that offer brain-stimulating benefits. This lesson discusses specific types of mental aerobics. As participants will learn, there are endless types of activities that are both fun and beneficial to the brain. The combination of thinking creatively, using your hands, meeting new people, and forcing your brain out of its "comfort zone" or normal circuitry is a recipe for improved brain health.

There are two broad categories of simple mental-aerobic activities that people can incorporate into daily life:

Do New Things. The brain is like a muscle. Just as the body gets used to exercising, the brain gets used to doing the same activities each day. While some routine in daily life is good, too much routine deprives the brain of the stimulation it needs to grow new nerve cells. For example, if you work on Sudoku puzzles at breakfast every morning and have found that they are not as challenging as when you first started working on the puzzles, try a different type of puzzle. Stimulating your brain in new and different ways is what causes new nerve cells to grow, which is the hallmark of the brain's ability to change and grow in response to learning (brain plasticity). This lesson will review a variety of activities that have been shown to enhance memory. Try something new today—you may just become hooked!

Do the Same Things, but Differently. Fortunately you don't have to go around filling your day with new activity after new activity to challenge your brain. You can also grow new nerve cells and challenge your brain by varying the way you do regular daily activities. For example, if you have driven the same route to the store for years, map out a new route for a change of scenery. Or try brushing your teeth or using your computer mouse with your opposite (nondominant) hand. Even something as simple as putting your clothes on in a different order can jolt your brain out of its comfort zone and help it to become stronger.

TYPES OF MENTAL AEROBICS

Word Puzzles. These pencil and paper puzzles, many of which can also be done via the Internet, have become extremely popular in recent years and are well known for their brain-boosting power. Examples include crossword puzzles, word searches, riddles, rebuses, Sudoku, trivia activities, and more. They are extremely good for challenging the brain and can help reduce cognitive decline, including "tip of the tongue" syndrome. In a study that involved individuals in their 70s and 80s who had mild cognitive impairment (MCI), those who played games (written or on the computer), read books, or engaged in creative activ-

ities were 30% to 50% less likely to develop memory loss than those who did not participate in these types of activities (Anderson, 2009).

Music. Numerous studies have documented the benefits of listening to music to enhance
memory. O'Brien (2000) reported on a study conducted by Bulgarian psychologist Georgi
Lozanov in the 1960s that found that people who listened to music while learning new
things were able to absorb the information better. In the experiment, some participants listened to slow Baroque music, while others studied in silence or listened to other types of
music. Lozanov found that the participants who listened to the Baroque music learned
better as compared to those who did not. Lozanov observed that "in certain circumstances
music can create an atmosphere that encourages mental absorption" (O'Brien, 2008, p. 86).

In another study involving people who had suffered a brain injury, researchers found
that those who had received musical training for between 1 and 5 years were able to recall
more words on a memory test than those who had not received musical training (Lavelle,
2003).

The so-called Mozart effect is when learning information and then recalling it is aided
by listening to the music of classical artist Amadeaus Mozart. According to O'Donnell
(1999), the music of Mozart has a 60 beats-per-minute pattern that activates the brain's left
side (which processes the information to be learned) and right side (which enhances retention), which maximizes learning and retention of information.

Clearly music is a powerful tool to enhance memory. Try to incorporate more music
into your daily life or even try testing the Mozart effect. Learn to play a new instrument,
which is especially beneficial because the left and right brain are used. Finally, remember
that to best enhance memory, music should complement an activity that you are engaged
in, not compete with it.

Reading. Reading is an excellent brain exercise. Boerner (n.d.) found a lower risk of dementia among those who read frequently. Reading stimulates the brain by forcing you to concentrate and process new concepts and ideas. If you were to join a book club, you would
double your brain workout by discussing the book with others. For maximum brain stimulation, try reading aloud. Doing so activates both sides of the brain, whereas reading to
yourself activates only one side.

Creativity. Many of the studies that have focused on mental aerobics and memory enhancement involve some component of creativity. A 2009 study called "Knitting Can Delay
Memory Loss" found that people who played games, read, or participated in craft hobbies
(patchworking, knitting) had a 40% reduced risk of memory impairment (BBC News,
2009). Unfortunately, the act of being creative is something that, throughout the working
years, many adults put aside. Even if you have never been an artistic or musical person,
there are plenty of ways to spark your inner creativity, including writing, painting, sketch-
ing, learning to play music, taking photographs, or doing needlework. Engaging in creative activities stimulates the right side of the brain, an area that most people use far less
than the left, more logical side.

Other Types of Activities. There are many other types of creative activities that offer brain
stimulating benefits:

- Learning another language is one of the most challenging activities to try because it
forces your brain to work extra hard, which means more mental stimulation and the
growth of more nerve cells in the long run.

- Acting is a wonderfully social activity that requires you to step into another person's
shoes and think like that person. It also forces you to meet new people and form new
relationships, both of which are great for improving brain health (more about this in
the class on Socialization).

- Playing board games such as Yahtzee, Scrabble, Pictionary, and Boggle activates the strategic, spatial, and memory parts of the brain (Boerner, n.d.), which can help form new nerve pathways. Joining a game group requires you to socialize, which also improves brain health.

- Find out what kind of classes your local junior college, adult school, or community center is offering. From tai chi to gardening to beadwork to writing, taking a class is a perfect way to expand your mental horizons.

Mental Aerobics
FACILITATOR INSTRUCTIONS

1. WELCOME AND INTRODUCTION (10 MINUTES)

To do before class:

- Read and familiarize yourself with the Mental Aerobics Overview.

- Write the following quotes on a board or flip chart.

> Music, when soft voices die, vibrates in the memory.
> (Percy Shelley, poet)

> A great and beautiful invention is memory, always useful both
> for learning and for life.
> (Greek Dialexeis)

- Have Mozart playing in the background as people arrive and take their seats.

- Familiarize yourself with and make appropriate copies of the warm-up activity, quiz, practice activities, and homework.

Greet the participants and tell them that the topic of the class will be mental aerobics. Ask them what types of activities come to mind when they think of the term *mental aerobics*. Is there any one kind of mental-aerobic activity that they think is better for the brain than another? Tell participants that a variety of activities that are good for the brain will be discussed as well as simple lifestyle changes that can help enhance memory. For example, explain how classical music, such as that by Mozart, can be beneficial for the brain.

Discuss the quotes and ask participants for their interpretations. Why do they think that playing or listening to music are such popular pastimes? Does anyone have a particular memory that is linked to a piece of music?

2. WARM-UP ACTIVITY (10 MINUTES)

For the group activity *Name 10 Things*, bring one of the following items to class with you: a paper clip, a small drinking cup, a thimble, or a roll of tape. Show the item to the class and ask them to spend a few minutes thinking of what the item could be used for. Encourage them to think creatively and outside the box. Silly answers are okay, too! After a few minutes, ask participants to share their answers. Then explain that this type of activity is an easy way to stimulate the brain and can easily be done with any type of object.

3.   MENTAL AEROBICS QUIZ (20 MINUTES)

Explain that the quiz for this lesson is not so much a test of knowledge as an assessment of how mentally active each participant is. Pass out the quiz and ask the class to read each statement and circle the number that best corresponds with their answer. Give about 5 to 10 minutes for everyone to finish and then ask them to add up (score) their answers. While participants are working, go around the room and ask if anyone has any questions or needs help adding up the answers. When everyone has finished, share with participants what the number totals mean. Ask if anyone would like to share how he or she did and if anyone was pleased with his or her score (or not).

4.   EXPLANATION AND DISCUSSION OF USING MENTAL AEROBICS FOR MEMORY ENHANCEMENT (10 MINUTES)

Discuss the two broad categories of mental aerobics that people can incorporate into their daily lives to enhance memory (*Do New Things*; *Do the Same Things, but Differently*). Take this time to review brain plasticity (that the brain can continue to learn new things no matter how much we age). Identify the different types of mental aerobics and their benefits and explain that participants will have a chance to try some of these activities in class.

5.   PRACTICE ACTIVITIES (30 MINUTES)

Distribute the worksheet *Name the States* and encourage participants to brainstorm and list as many of the 50 states as they can. Try to have a blank map available to help provide a visual cue for thinking of as many states as possible. After about 10 minutes, ask participants how they did. Did anyone get all 50 states? Did anyone use any special technique to help remember the states (using the alphabet, working region by region or coast to coast, listing states that they have been to)?

Pass out the worksheet *Cultivating Creativity* and explain that even though someone may not think of him- or herself as a creative person, everyone has the ability to become more creative. Ask participants to close their eyes and think of three of their favorite places. Then ask them to write 10 words that describe each place. Encourage them to think of what this place is like from the perspective of each of their five senses. After everyone has finished, ask if anyone would like to share one of their favorite places and what it is like.

Hand out the list *Using Mental Aerobics in Everyday Life* and explain that we can do many activities in everyday life that have brain-stimulating benefits. Read and discuss the list with participants and ask if any one activity stands out as something that each might like to try. Encourage participants to post the list at home where it can be easily seen and they can refer to it regularly for quick and easy brain-stimulating activities to do in their everyday lives.

6.   REVIEW AND CLOSING (5 MINUTES)

Thank the participants for coming to class and express your hope that they had fun taking part in some mentally simulating activities and in learning about the importance of keeping the mind active. Review the importance of trying new activities as well as doing routine things in new ways. Ask participants to think about at least one new activity that they will incorporate into their routines this week.

7.   HOMEWORK (5 MINUTES)

Pass out the homework sheets, explain what should be done for each, and encourage everyone to complete them during the week. Remind them that homework should be fun and suggest that they enlist the help of family and friends, if they can.

- *Numbers, Numbers, Numbers*

- *The Sound of Music*

- Try at least one new mental aerobics activity this week!

Mental Aerobics
CLASS AGENDA

1. Welcome and Introduction
2. Warm-Up Activity
   - *Name 10 Things* (Group Activity)
3. Mental Aerobics Quiz
4. Overview of Mental Aerobics for Memory Enhancement
   - Two broad types of mental aerobics
   - Specific types of mental aerobics
5. Practice Activities
   - *Name the States*
   - *Cultivating Creativity*
   - *Using Mental Aerobics in Everyday Life*
6. Review and Closing
7. Homework
   - *Numbers, Numbers, Numbers,*
   - *The Sound of Music*
   - Try at least one new mental aerobics activity this week!

Strengthen Your Mind Program: A Course for Memory Enhancement by Einberger & Sellick.

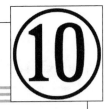

Name 10 Things

Other than its intended purpose, what could the object be used for?
Silly, senseless, and out of the ordinary answers are welcome!

1.

2.

3.

4.

5.

6.

7.

8.

9.

10.

Strengthen Your Mind Program: A Course for Memory Enhancement by Einberger & Sellick.
© 2010 by Health Professions Press, Inc.

Mental Aerobics Quiz

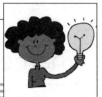

How mentally active are you? Read the statements below and circle the number that best fits your answer. If there is an activity that you have not participated in at all in the past year, then do not circle any number. When you are finished, add your numbers together to get a total.

	At least once in the past year	At least once in the past month	At least once in the past week
1. Worked on a crossword puzzle	1	2	3
2. Read a book	1	2	3
3. Listened to music	1	2	3
4. Spoke or tried to learn another language	1	2	3
5. Tried a new food	1	2	3
6. Put together a jigsaw puzzle	1	2	3
7. Engaged in a spirited discussion with others	1	2	3
8. Took a walk outside	1	2	3
9. Participated in a volunteer activity	1	2	3
10. Met a new friend	1	2	3
11. Taught (or explained) to someone how to do something	1	2	3
12. Played brain games on the computer	1	2	3
13. Attended a seminar, reading, or other event	1	2	3
14. Played a board game, such as Scrabble or Yahtzee	1	2	3
15. Rearranged or redesigned an area in your home	1	2	3
16. Played a musical instrument	1	2	3
17. Participated in a creative activity, such as knitting, woodworking, or painting	1	2	3
18. Tried a new hobby or pastime	1	2	3
19. Took time to "stop and smell the roses"	1	2	3
20. Sketched, painted, or doodled	1	2	3
21. Worked math problems	1	2	3
Add numbers together for total	_____	_____	_____

Strengthen Your Mind Program: A Course for Memory Enhancement by Einberger & Sellick.

Mental Aerobics Quiz ANSWER SHEET

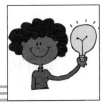

How did participants do on the quiz? Ask them to total their numbers from each column (add them together) and then add the numbers from the three columns together to get a grand total.

Score:

0–20   Oh dear! Your brain is crying out for some mental stimulation! Start right away by picking an activity you might enjoy and trying it, even if just for 10 minutes a few times a week. Or, vary your daily routine so that your brain gets a jump start from mental activity.

21–41   Good job! You have been spending time participating in healthy, mentally stimulating activities. Hopefully you have noticed an improvement in the clarity of your thinking and an overall feeling of well-being as a result. Now is the time to step up your involvement and try something new.

42–63   Excellent! You are a brain health pro! By regularly making an effort to participate in mentally stimulating activities, you are constantly growing new nerve cells and making new connections in your brain, both of which contribute to better memory and thinking. Keep up the good work and remember not to let your activities get too routine.

Strengthen Your Mind Program: A Course for Memory Enhancement by Einberger & Sellick.
© 2010 by Health Professions Press, Inc.

Name the States

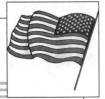

List as many of the 50 states as you can, and don't worry if you can't name them all!

1.	26.
2.	27.
3.	28.
4.	29.
5.	30.
6.	31.
7.	32.
8.	33.
9.	34.
10.	35.
11.	36.
12.	37.
13.	38.
14.	39.
15.	40.
16.	41.
17.	42.
18.	43.
19.	44.
20.	45.
21.	46.
22.	47.
23.	48.
24.	49.
25.	50.

Name the States ANSWER SHEET

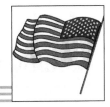

Alabama	Montana
Alaska	Nebraska
Arizona	Nevada
Arkansas	New Hampshire
California	New Jersey
Colorado	New Mexico
Connecticut	New York
Delaware	North Carolina
Florida	North Dakota
Georgia	Ohio
Hawaii	Oklahoma
Idaho	Oregon
Illinois	Pennsylvania
Indiana	Rhode Island
Iowa	South Carolina
Kansas	South Dakota
Kentucky	Tennessee
Louisiana	Texas
Maine	Utah
Maryland	Vermont
Massachusetts	Virginia
Michigan	Washington
Minnesota	West Virginia
Mississippi	Wisconsin
Missouri	Wyoming

Cultivating Creativity

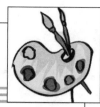

Think of three favorite places that you have been to or would like to go to. List them below and use 10 adjectives to describe each. Try to imagine what each place is like using each of your senses.

Place #1 _____

Descriptive Words

Place #2 _____

Descriptive Words

Place #3 _____

Descriptive Words

Strengthen Your Mind Program: A Course for Memory Enhancement by Einberger & Sellick.

Using Mental Aerobics in Everyday Life

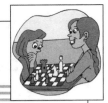

We can do many activities in everyday life that have brain-stimulating benefits. Below are several examples. Try at least one new mental aerobic activity each week!

1. Spend time in a new environment, store, park, or museum that you have never been to before.

2. Try brushing your teeth or using the computer mouse with your nondominant hand.

3. Find a new route to a friend's house, to a store, to church, and so forth.

4. Distinguish coins using only your sense of touch.

5. Vary the order in which you perform your daily routine.

6. Read something completely different from what you usually read.

7. Discuss politics, trends, history, and so forth with friends.

8. Communicate a thought or idea to someone without using your voice.

9. Try a new board game with friends.

10. Say the alphabet backwards.

11. Close your eyes as you [shower], and use your sense of touch to locate your [shampoo]. (Fill in the brackets with other activities.)

12. Learn to write your name with your nondominant hand.

13. Learn three phrases in another language.

14. Rearrange the furniture in a room or in your entire home.

15. Volunteer to read aloud to kids at a library.

16. Learn one new type of dance.

17. If you're the passenger in a car, train, bus, plane, or so forth, bring word search or crossword puzzles with you.

18. Practice memorizing your errand list instead of writing it down.

19. Join or create a trivia club.

20. Try the crossword puzzle in the Sunday (or daily) newspaper.

Strengthen Your Mind Program: A Course for Memory Enhancement by Einberger & Sellick.
© 2010 by Health Professions Press, Inc.

Numbers, Numbers, Numbers

Each phrase below has a corresponding number. How many do you know?

1. Letters of the alphabet
2. Wonders of the world
3. Signs of the zodiac
4. Cards in a deck (with jokers)
5. Planets in the solar system
6. Piano keys
7. Baker's dozen
8. Holes on a golf course
9. Degrees in a right angle
10. Sides of a stop sign
11. Quarts in a gallon
12. Hours in a day
13. Wheels on a unicycle
14. Varieties of Heinz products
15. Players on a football team (on the field)
16. Words that a picture is worth
17. Squares on a checkerboard
18. Days and nights of the Great Flood
19. Leagues under the sea
20. Digits in a social security number
21. Jack Benny's age
22. Number of black birds baked in a pie
23. Yards in a soccer field
24. Countries in North America
25. The world's major oceans
26. Continents in the world
27. Senators in the U.S. Senate
28. Representatives in the U.S. House of Representatives

Strengthen Your Mind Program: A Course for Memory Enhancement by Einberger & Sellick.

Numbers, Numbers, Numbers ANSWER SHEET

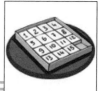

1.	Letters of the alphabet	**26**
2.	Wonders of the world	**7**
3.	Signs of the zodiac	**12**
4.	Cards in a deck (with jokers)	**54**
5.	Planets in the solar system	**8 (previously 9)**
6.	Piano keys	**88**
7.	Baker's dozen	**13**
8.	Holes on a golf course	**18**
9.	Degrees in a right angle	**90**
10.	Sides of a stop sign	**8**
11.	Quarts in a gallon	**4**
12.	Hours in a day	**24**
13.	Wheels on a unicycle	**1**
14.	Varieties of Heinz products	**57**
15.	Players on a football team (on the field)	**11**
16.	Words that a picture is worth	**1,000**
17.	Squares on a checkerboard	**64**
18.	Days and nights of the Great Flood	**40**
19.	Leagues under the sea	**20,000**
20.	Digits in a social security number	**9**
21.	Jack Benny's age	**39**
22.	Number of black birds baked in a pie	**4 and 20**
23.	Yards in a soccer field	**100 (can be up to 130)**
24.	Countries in North America	**23 (including islands)**
25.	The world's major oceans	**5**
26.	Continents in the world	**7**
27.	Senators in the U.S. Senate	**100**
28.	Representatives in the U.S. House of Representatives	**435**

The Sound of Music

Webster's Dictionary defines *music* as vocal, instrumental, or mechanical sounds having rhythm, melody, or harmony. For most of us, music is an integral part of our lives, whether by listening, playing, singing, or composing. The following questions relate to music in a variety of ways. How many can you answer?

1.   Which stringed instrument is commonly used in bluegrass music?

2.   How many types of music can you name?

3.   This pluck-stringed, usually triangular-shaped instrument is said to be played by angels floating on clouds. Its strings are perpendicular to the soundboard.

4.   This musical instrument, played on a keyboard, is often used for accompaniment. One of the most popular types is the Baby Grand.

5.   This boogie-woogie, ragtime style of music is played on the instrument described in question number 4.

6.   Many churches have one of these, which consists of sets of pipes.

7.   The most popular music lessons taken by children are with this instrument.

8.   This classification of musical instruments, often used to accompany, includes the drums, tambourines, bells, cymbals, and congas.

9.   This group of four people sings harmoniously without musical accompaniment. The group often wears colorful outfits, bow ties, and boater hats.

10. This stringed instrument in the violin family was first crafted by a famous Italian family in the 1600s and represents a high standard of excellence. Jack Benny often used it in his comedy routine.

11. This Austrian capital is one of the great music cities of the world.

12. This southern U.S. city is often said to be the birthplace of jazz.

13. The Grand Ole Opry in this town is the center of country music.

14. How many string instruments can you name?

Reprinted from *Strengthen Your Mind, Volume Two* by Einberger & Sellick.
© 2008 by Health Professions Press, Inc.

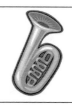

1. Which stringed instrument is commonly used in bluegrass music?
   banjo or mandolin

2. How many types of music can you name?
   opera, folk, rock and roll, country, western, rap, jazz, blues, religious, flamenco, orchestra, marching band, and so forth.

3. This pluck-stringed, usually triangular-shaped instrument is said to be played by angels floating on clouds. Its strings are perpendicular to the soundboard.
   harp

4. This musical instrument, played on a keyboard, is often used for accompaniment. One of the most popular types is the Baby Grand.
   piano

5. This boogie-woogie, ragtime style of music is played on the instrument described in question number 4.
   honky-tonk

6. Many churches have one of these, which consists of sets of pipes.
   organ

7. The most popular music lessons taken by children are with this instrument.
   piano

8. This classification of musical instruments, often used to accompany, includes the drums, tambourines, bells, cymbals, and congas.
   percussion

9. This group of four people sings harmoniously without musical accompaniment. The group often wears colorful outfits, bow ties, and boater hats.
   barbershop quartet

10. This stringed instrument in the violin family was first crafted by a famous Italian family in the 1600s and represents a high standard of excellence. Jack Benny often used it in his comedy routine.
    Stradivarius

11. This Austrian capital is one of the great music cities of the world.
    Vienna

12. This southern U.S. city is often said to be the birthplace of jazz.
    New Orleans

13. The Grand Ole Opry in this town is the center of country music.
    Nashville

14. How many string instruments can you name?
    violin, viola, harp, guitar, cello, bass, harpsichord, lute, mandolin, ukulele, dulcimer, autoharp, and so forth.

Exercise

Exercise
FACILITATOR OVERVIEW

Exercise has long been touted as some of the best preventive medicine to be found. Indeed, regular physical activity can stave off some of the most devastating diseases that our society faces. What about exercise and memory? What effect does regular exercise have on a person's cognitive function? As part of this lesson participants will learn about three types of exercise and how each affects brain function. They will also learn about how much exercise is necessary for improved well-being and discuss ways to include more exercise in their everyday lives.

TYPES OF EXERCISE

There are three main types of exercise that, when done in moderation, can benefit the body and mind. The first type, cardiovascular exercise, causes your heart to pump blood faster throughout your body. You may feel out of breath, break a sweat, or feel tired after cardiovascular exercise. Examples are brisk walking, swimming, jogging, bicycling, and playing tennis. The benefits of cardiovascular exercise are a lower heart rate, lower blood pressure, improved physical fitness, and a faster metabolism (which means that your body burns more calories even while at rest!). The good thing about cardiovascular exercise is that you can do it almost anywhere. Any exercise that gets your heart pumping faster for a period of time is considered cardiovascular exercise.

The second type of exercise that is beneficial is strength or resistance training, including lifting weights, yoga, pilates, and any exercise that uses natural or artificial resistance. Strength training may cause your muscles to feel tired and possibly even sore afterward. The benefits of strength training, however, are endless, especially for older adults. Strength training keeps the muscles strong and toned, which makes you feel and look better! Resistance exercises also make the bones stronger, which reduces the likelihood of developing osteoporosis or experiencing a bone fracture. Finally, strength and resistance training improve balance, coordination, and posture, all of which can make you feel better about yourself.

Stretching and flexibility are the third type of exercise. Stretching is when a specific muscle (or muscle group) is elongated to its fullest length. Stretching increases flexibility, enhances the range of motion of joints, decreases the likelihood of pulling or tearing a muscle, improves circulation, and can relieve stress. Flexibility is the ability to move joints and muscles through their full range of motion. Flexibility exercises are excellent for improving balance and posture. Examples of stretching and flexibility include rotating your joints (arm circles), trying to touch your toes (always with your knees slightly bent to protect your lower back!), reaching your arms above your head, swinging your arms back and forth, and twisting your torso from side to side. Stretching exercises are especially important as you grow older because they counteract the natural decline in flexibility that all of us experience as we age. When you stretch you may feel a pulling sensation in your muscles, and if you stretch too far, it may hurt, so make sure to start out slowly. Stretching can easily be done anywhere. You can increase your flexibility while watching television, talking on the phone, folding laundry, or working in the kitchen. You don't need any special equipment, just the desire to keep your body flexible and healthy.

BENEFITS OF EXERCISE ON COGNITIVE FUNCTION

Exercise is an important part of a healthy lifestyle, but how exactly does it affect memory? One of the most significant studies in recent years found that people age 50 and older who walked for the equivalent of 2½ hours each week performed better on cognitive tests, had lower clinical dementia scores, and had better recall (Lautenschlager et al., 2008). The study was led by researchers at the University of Melbourne and found that the cognitive benefits of the exercise program lasted for at least a year after completion of the supervised physical activity program. The good news is that walking 2½ hours each week can be broken down into 30 minutes 5 days a week or an hour twice a week and half an hour once a week—a feasible amount of time for most people.

An additional study found that women age 65 and older who took part in regular exercise had cognitive function scores 10% higher than their peers who did not exercise (McKeever, 2009). According to the author of the study, Marc Poulin, "Being sedentary is now considered a risk factor for stroke and dementia." Finally, in a study of the effects of exercise and fitness on people older than age 60 and with early Alzheimer's disease, those who had higher physical fitness ratings had less atrophy in key areas associated with memory (Basler, 2008). The findings of the study, which compared the brains of 56 healthy people with 63 people who had early Alzheimer's disease and who were not as physically fit, suggest that cardiovascular exercise may help modify, slow down the progress of, or even correct some of the damage that Alzheimer's disease causes in the brain.

One theory as to why cardiovascular exercise benefits cognitive function is that it helps maintain blood flow to the brain as people age. And, according to McKeever (2009), "Better blood flow translates into improved cognition."

Strength- and resistance-training exercises have been proven to help memory as well. One study examined the effects of resistance training on well-being and memory in 46 volunteers with an average age of 73. Participants in the study took part in an 8-week resistance-training program that involved a 10-minute warm-up followed by 8 resistance exercises on machines (Perrig-Chiello et al., 1998). This study found that participants' memory recall and recognition were improved and were still improved even a year later.

Although few studies have focused specifically on the cognitive benefits of stretching, regular stretching and flexibility exercises can help to keep the brain's arteries open and unclogged. Making a habit of stretching can also boost energy, increase flexibility, and improve attitude, all of which contribute to better long-term memory. In addition, being flexible can make it easier to do many daily activities, which increases the sense of independence and youthfulness, which, in turn, improve well-being and mental health.

The following is a summary of the benefits of exercise on memory. People who exercise regularly:

- Perform better on cognitive function tests

- Multitask better

- Score lower on tests that measure signs of dementia

- Benefit from improved cognitive function that lasts for at least a year after starting an exercise routine or program

- Improve memory recall and recognition

- May reduce the risk of developing dementia

- May succeed in slowing the progression of memory-related illnesses

HOW TO INCORPORATE EXERCISE INTO EVERYDAY LIFE

It can be difficult to fit exercise into everyday life, especially for people who have never enjoyed physical fitness before. One of the most important things to remember is that exercise can be fun and endless varieties of exercise can meet most individuals' interests. Even for people who are avid fitness buffs, there is always room to make an exercise program more well rounded. Most people who exercise regularly, for example, do not take enough time to stretch. Others do plenty of cardiovascular exercise throughout the week but rarely take time to do any strength-training exercises. All three types of exercise are important for a healthy mind and body.

Below are ideas for how to incorporate each type of exercise into daily life. Getting into the habit of exercising takes some practice, but small steps add up to big results! When you do exercise, make a mental note of how good you feel all over for the next time you need a little motivation to lace up those shoes. Your mind and your body will thank you!

Cardiovascular Exercises. Find a walking buddy. Start by walking around the block and gradually increase the distance that you walk. Join a gym and take cardiovascular classes, walk on the treadmill, or use the stationary bike. Park your car farther away and walk the extra distance (it all adds up!). Even better, walk to your destination instead of driving. Develop a new hobby by signing up for a class, such as swimming, tennis, or biking. Most local community or senior centers offer classes specifically for adults older than age 50. Play tag with your grandchildren. Take your dog (or someone else's!) for a walk. Take up dancing with your partner or a friend or try water aerobics.

Strength- or Resistance-Training Exercises. Any exercise that works against the force of gravity is a strength-training or weight-bearing exercise. Try a pilates class or buy a set of weights and lift for 10 minutes a day. Climb the stairs instead of taking the elevator. Pull weeds in the garden. Go canoeing or kayaking. Take a weight-training class at the gym. Carry your groceries out to your car in a bag instead of using a cart. Walk or jog (both cardiovascular and strength training). Buy or borrow a resistance band and use it while you watch television. Do push-ups against the wall.

Stretching and Flexibility Exercises. Try a new class, such as tai chi or yoga. Stretch while you watch television. Move your wrists around in circles while you are at a red light. Take a 5-minute stretch break morning, noon, and night. Reach up to the ceiling when you first wake up in the morning.

Exercise
FACILITATOR INSTRUCTIONS

1. WELCOME AND INTRODUCTION (10 MINUTES)

To do before class:

- Read and familiarize yourself with the Exercise Overview.

- Write the following quotes on a board or flip chart.

> "Movement is a medicine for creating change in a person's physical, emotional, and mental states."
> (Carol Welch, author)

> "It is exercise alone that supports the spirits, and keeps the mind in vigor."
> (Marcus Tullius Cicero, Roman philosopher)

- Familiarize yourself with and make appropriate copies of the warm-up activity, quiz, practice activities, and homework.

Greet the participants and make introductions, if necessary. Explain that the topic of the class is exercise and how it benefits memory. Ask how many people make an effort to exercise regularly. Explain that as we grow older one of the most important things that we can do for our bodies and minds is to keep moving.

Discuss the quotes and ask participants for their interpretations. Ask what types of exercise they enjoy doing and how often. How do they feel, both physically and mentally, after working out?

2. WARM-UP ACTIVITY (10 MINUTES)

Pass out the *Exercise A–Z* worksheet and explain that it will help participants think about the broad scope and variety of exercises that can be done. Remind them that it is great to think outside the box and to be creative when listing the different exercises.

3. EXERCISE QUIZ (10 MINUTES)

Hand out the Exercise Quiz and give participants about 5 minutes to complete it. Remind everyone that it's alright if they don't know all of the answers and to just do the best that they can. After everyone has finished, review the quiz by talking about each answer one by one, pausing for questions and comments. Ask participants how they did and explain that the class will teach them more about exercise and how it affects the body and mind.

4. EXPLANATION AND DISCUSSION OF EXERCISE AND HOW IT AFFECTS MEMORY (15 MINUTES)

Discuss each type of exercise and how important each is in maintaining overall fitness and health. Write each type of exercise (cardiovascular, strength training, stretching and flexibility) on a board or flip chart, and ask participants to brainstorm types of exercise that are appropriate for each category. Review the findings of the studies mentioned in the overview and emphasize that exercise really does benefit the mind as well as the body.

5. PRACTICE ACTIVITIES (30 MINUTES)

Explain that it is often difficult to stay motivated and exercise regularly. The most benefits, however, can be gained when exercise is made a regular part of life instead of starting and stopping a fitness routine or program many times. Invite participants to break up into three smaller groups (you can count off 1, 2, 3 or divide them up how you choose).

Pass out the worksheets *Overcoming Fitness Barriers* (one for each of the three types of exercise). Give one group the worksheet for cardiovascular exercises, another group the one for strength training exercises, and the third group the worksheet for stretching and flexibility exercises. Ask each group to work together to complete the worksheet and brainstorm answers to the questions. Give the groups about 10 minutes. When they have finished, ask one person from each group to talk about the exercise challenges and successes that people in the group have experienced, the exercises that they have done or are currently doing, and their ideas for other exercises that they could do.

Explain that the class will now discuss some more ideas for overcoming barriers and staying motivated to exercise.

Distribute the handout *10 Tips for Staying Motivated!* Read aloud each of the points listed. Use the answer sheet provided for this handout to explain each point, pausing for questions and comments. Sample questions to encourage discussion include: "Would this tip help you to stay motivated?" "Have you ever tried this method?" "How would you modify or change this tip to work for you?"

Explain that the class will now practice a memory-enhancement technique that involves movement.

Pass out the worksheet *Using Motor Cues to Remember Names*. Explain to the class that research has shown that people learn and remember information better if they incorporate movement. A person can use the technique of using a motor cue to remember a name by creating a movement that corresponds with an activity that he or she enjoys. For example, if Bob enjoys fishing, his motor cue might be moving his hands as if casting out a line. Have the group practice saying the name "Bob" while moving as if they were casting out a fishing line.

Each participant will next create a motor cue for him- or herself. Ask participants to think of one activity or hobby that they especially enjoy. Ask them to then think of a movement that corresponds with the activity or hobby. (While they are writing on the worksheet, go around and ask if anyone needs help coming up with an idea.) When each person has finished, ask everyone to stand up and then go around the room and have each person say his or her name and make the motion of his or her motor cue. (Depending on the size of the class, you may ask everyone to share or, if the class is especially large, only a few.) Ask the rest of the group to get involved by repeating the person's name and making the motion of his or her motor cue. You may go around the room a few times to practice the motor cues. Explain to the group that as part of the next class on Strategies for Memory Improvement they will try this exercise again and will see how beneficial moving the body is while trying to remember something.

6. REVIEW AND CLOSING (10 MINUTES)

Thank the group for their participation in the class and encourage them to try at least one new exercise this week. Remind them that exercise is vital to physical and mental health and at any age—20, 50, or 90 years old! Review the benefits of exercise on memory. Ask participants to take a moment to think about one new exercise that they could incorporate into their daily routine this week.

7. HOMEWORK (5 MINUTES)

Pass out the homework sheets, explain what should be done for each, and encourage everyone to complete them during the week. Remind them that homework should be fun and suggest that they enlist the help of family and friends, if they can.

- *Athletes of Greatness*

- *Exercise Puzzle*

- Pump up your exercise routine by adding cardiovascular, strength training, or stretching and flexibility exercises—whichever you could use more of!

Exercise
CLASS AGENDA

1. Welcome and Introduction
2. Warm-Up Activity
   - *Exercise A–Z*
3. Exercise Quiz
4. Overview of Exercise and How It Affects Memory
   - Types of Exercise
   - How Does Exercise Affect the Brain?
   - Incorporating Exercise into Everyday Life
5. Practice Activities
   - *Overcoming Fitness Barriers*
   - *10 Tips for Staying Motivated!*
   - *Using Motor Cues to Remember Names*
6. Review and Closing
7. Homework
   - *Athletes of Greatness*
   - *Exercise Puzzle*
   - Pump up your exercise routine!

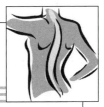

Exercise A–Z

List a type of exercise that begins with each letter of the alphabet. Be creative!

A

B

C

D

E

F

G

H

I

J

K

L

M

N

O

P

Q

R

S

T

U

V

W

X

Y

Z

Exercise Quiz

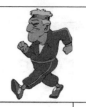

1. Exercise that gets the heart pumping faster is called what?
    A. sweating exercise
    B. cardiovascular exercise
    C. cardiopulmonary respiration
    D. a workout for the heart

2. True or False? When considering a fitness program, the only exercise you really need to do regularly is cardiovascular.

3. Which of the following will not help to strengthen bones and prevent osteoporosis?
    A. lifting weights
    B. walking
    C. swimming
    D. tennis

4. True or False? Exercise can be just as effective as medication for preventing depression in older adults.

5. Which of the following will not help to improve flexibility?
    A. yoga
    B. weight lifting
    C. stretching
    D. pilates

6. How many hours of exercise should you do each week to benefit your mind and body?
    A. 1½
    B. 2½
    C. 5
    D. 7

7. True or False? Stretching exercises should be performed before and after doing cardiovascular or strength-training exercises.

Strengthen Your Mind Program: A Course for Memory Enhancement by Einberger & Sellick.
© 2010 by Health Professions Press, Inc.

8. Which disease usually makes it impossible to take part in a regular exercise program?
   A. high blood pressure
   B. diabetes
   C. obesity
   D. arthritis
   E. none of the above

9. Which of the following exercises can help you feel more alert?
   A. weight lifting
   B. walking
   C. stretching
   D. all of the above
   E. none of the above

10. True or False? Engaging in a regular exercise program can help reduce the risk of developing dementia.

Exercise Quiz ANSWER SHEET

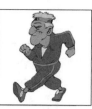

1. **Exercise that gets the heart pumping faster is called what?**

    B. cardiovascular exercise. Also called *aerobic exercise,* cardiovascular exercise is an excellent way to fight heart disease, burn calories, and keep your brain sharp.

2. **True or False? When considering a fitness program, the only exercise you really need to do regularly is cardiovascular.**

    False. Cardiovascular exercise is an excellent way to start a fitness program. A well-rounded program, however, should incorporate stretching and strength-training exercises as well.

3. **Which of the following will not help to strengthen bones and prevent osteoporosis?**

    C. swimming. Your body is buoyant in water, which takes away the effect of gravity. Weight-bearing exercises work against the force of gravity, thereby building strength.

4. **True or False? Exercise can be just as effective as medication for preventing depression in older adults.**

    True. Exercise is an all-natural mood booster and can be as effective as medication in preventing depression.

5. **Which of the following will not help to improve flexibility?**

    B. weight lifting. Although an excellent exercise to strengthen muscles, weight lifting will not make them more flexible.

6. **How many hours of exercise should you do each week to benefit your mind and body?**

    B. 2½. At a minimum, aim for half an hour five times a week. One hour five times a week is even better!

7. **True or False? Stretching exercises should be performed before and after doing cardiovascular or strength-training exercises.**

    True. Stretching is a great way to warm up and cool down. Just make sure that you don't stretch your muscles too far before you have exercised.

Strengthen Your Mind Program: A Course for Memory Enhancement by Einberger & Sellick.
© 2010 by Health Professions Press, Inc.

8. **Which disease usually makes it impossible to take part in a regular exercise program?**

   E. none of the above. With a doctor's approval, exercise can help to combat the effects of all of the diseases.

9. **Which of the following exercises can help you feel more alert?**

   D. all of the above. All three types of exercise improve blood flow to the brain, which can make you feel more alert and awake.

10. **True or False? Engaging in a regular exercise program can help reduce the risk of developing dementia.**

    True. Studies have shown that regular exercise can help keep the body and mind sharp and reduce the likelihood of developing dementia.

Overcoming Fitness Barriers

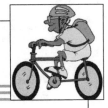

Cardiovascular Exercise

1. What types of cardiovascular exercise do you do now?

2. What are some other cardiovascular exercises that you could (or would like to) incorporate into your exercise program?

3. What are some barriers that prevent you from doing cardiovascular exercise as often as you would like?

4. How can you overcome or modify some of these barriers?

5. In general, what motivates you to exercise?

Strengthen Your Mind Program: A Course for Memory Enhancement by Einberger & Sellick.

Overcoming Fitness Barriers

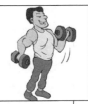

Strength-Training Exercise

1. What types of strength-training exercise do you do now?

2. What are some other strength-training exercises that you could (or would like to) incorporate into your exercise program?

3. What are some barriers that prevent you from doing strength-training exercise as often as you would like?

4. How can you overcome or modify some of these barriers?

5. In general, what motivates you to exercise?

Overcoming Fitness Barriers

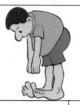

Stretching and Flexibility Exercises

1. What types of stretching and flexibility exercises do you do now?

2. What are some other stretching and flexibility exercises that you could (or would like to) incorporate into your exercise program?

3. What are some barriers that prevent you from doing stretching and flexibility exercises as often as you would like?

4. How can you overcome or modify some of these barriers?

5. In general, what motivates you to exercise?

Strengthen Your Mind Program: A Course for Memory Enhancement by Einberger & Sellick.

10 Tips for Staying Motivated!

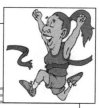

The "motivation blues" can hit any of us at any time. Below are some tips to encourage you to stay active and incorporate more exercise into your life.

1. Watch your words.

2. Commit to 10 minutes.

3. Start slowly.

4. Put yourself first.

5. Write down your reasons for exercising.

6. Create a goal.

7. Be flexible.

8. Include a buddy.

9. Reward yourself.

10. Have fun!

10 Tips for Staying Motivated! ANSWER SHEET

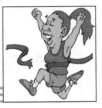

1. **Watch your words.**
    Reframe how you talk about exercise. Instead of "I have to go to the gym," try "I want to go to the aerobics class at the gym this afternoon." Or, instead of "I have to exercise more," practice saying "I want to exercise more."

2. **Commit to 10 minutes.**
    Often the hardest part of getting out the door to exercise is just that—getting out the door. Tell yourself that you only need to do 10 minutes of walking (or whatever exercise you prefer), and usually once you get started you won't want to stop.

3. **Start slowly.**
    When you first begin a new exercise give yourself (and your muscles) time to adjust. If you push yourself too hard in the beginning, you may feel sore and miserable for the next time. It is better to pace yourself and really enjoy what you are doing.

4. **Put yourself first.**
    Some people view taking time to exercise as selfish because it takes time away from family obligations or work. Remind yourself that you need to take care of yourself first before you can be there for others. Or, sign up for an event for a cause. Many programs will help you train for a walking, running, bicycle, or other event while you raise funds in support of an important charity. You'll help yourself while helping others!

5. **Write down your reasons for exercising.**
    Putting something down on paper always makes it more concrete. Write down all of the reasons that you want to begin or expand your exercise program. Revisit this list when you need motivation.

6. **Create a goal.**
    Completing a 5-kilometer walk, reaching to touch your toes, being able to do 5 push-ups—setting a goal that is clear and attainable will help motivate you as well as help you to keep track of your progress.

7. **Be flexible.**
    Life gets hectic and sometimes things get too busy for you to stick with your original plan. Don't beat yourself up if you can't get your workout in. If you had planned to go for a swim, instead try fitting in a quick walk. Remember that doing something is better than nothing and just get back into the swing of things the next day.

 Strengthen Your Mind Program: A Course for Memory Enhancement by Einberger & Sellick.

8. Include a buddy.

It's much easier to stick with an exercise routine if you have someone to work out with, even if it's just part of the time. Ask around for a walking buddy or someone with whom you can chat about your progress. Sharing with others is a real motivator.

9. Reward yourself.

Be proud of the changes you have made in your lifestyle, and take time to savor the great feeling that you get after exercising. Reward yourself for sticking with your plan (e.g., a night out at the movies after the first week of exercise).

10. Have fun!

It is hard to stick with something that is not enjoyable to you. Make sure that you are enjoying any exercise that you do. If swimming is not as enjoyable as you had thought, instead try joining a softball league or doing water aerobics. Incorporate fun little bits of exercise throughout your day. For example, play with your (or a neighbor's) pet, collect leaves, garden, or go for a walk on the beach. Mixing things up does wonders for motivation.

Using Motor Cues to Remember Names

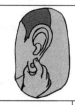

Using a motor cue to learn and remember new information involves creating a movement that corresponds with an activity or hobby that you enjoy. Follow the directions below to create a motor cue for your own name.

1. List an activity or hobby that you enjoy.

2. Create a body movement that corresponds with the activity or hobby (e.g., hands opening a book to signify reading).

3. Practice saying your name while making the body movement.

4. Go around the room and practice other people's names and motor cues. See how well you are able to remember their names!

List other class member's motor cues below.

Name: _____ Motor Cue: _____

Name: _____ Motor Cue: _____

Name: _____ Motor Cue: _____

Name: _____ Motor Cue: _____

Name: _____ Motor Cue: _____

Strengthen Your Mind Program: A Course for Memory Enhancement by Einberger & Sellick.

Athletes of Greatness

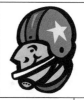

From the ancient Olympics, which began in 776 BC, to the modern Olympic games, which began in 1896, people have shown a great interest in watching sports and have revered great athletes. The truly great athletes often become "household names," even for those who are not particularly interested in the sport. Below are some facts regarding some of the most famous athletes of the last 100 years. Can you name them?

1. In 1926, this American female swimmer became the first woman to swim across the English Channel. Upon returning home, she received a very large ticker-tape parade in New York City.

2. This man, nicknamed "The Greatest," "The Champ," and "Louisville Lip," was one of the best heavyweight boxers of all time. He changed his birth name when he was a young man after he converted to Islam.

3. This runner won gold medals in both the decathlon and the pentathlon. He also excelled in many other sports, including football, baseball, and basketball. Being of mixed Native American and white ancestry, he struggled with racism throughout his sports career.

4. This great swimmer won an unprecedented seven events—all that he entered—in the 1972 summer Olympics in Germany.

5. Perhaps the most famous baseball player of all time, this New York Yankee "Sultan of Swat" held the home run record of 60 in a season, until Roger Maris broke it in the early 1960s. He changed the game of baseball with his power and his personality.

6. In 1947, this Brooklyn Dodger great became the first black major league baseball player in modern times. Inducted into the Hall of Fame in 1962, he was a member of six World Series winning teams and also won many other awards.

7. This man, one of the greatest golfers of all time, was nicknamed "The King." He won seven major championships between 1958 and 1964 and continued to play professionally until 2004.

8. This 7'1" basketball player was nicknamed " . . . the Stilt." He is the only player to average more than 50 points per game in a season and also the only one to score a whopping 100 points in a single game!

9. This female swimmer wrote an autobiography named *The Million Dollar Mermaid*. She went on from swimming to become a very successful movie star of the 1940s and '50s.

10. This world famous bike rider won an unprecedented seven consecutive Tour de France road races from 1999 to 2005. After courageously beating cancer, he began a foundation to fight the disease. His yellow "Live Strong" rubber bracelets have become popular throughout the world and have raised many millions of dollars to support his foundation.

11. This child prodigy began playing golf at age 2 and by age 8 was winning tournaments. In 2006, he was the highest paid athlete, winning $100 million in tournaments and endorsements! He has been the PGA Player of the Year eight times.

12. This football great spent most of his years as quarterback for the New York Jets, beginning in 1965. His antics, both on and off the field, were legendary. He appeared in many advertisements and was especially known for Remington electric shaver ads. His nickname is "Broadway . . ."

Athletes of Greatness ANSWER SHEET

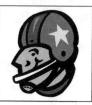

1. In 1926, this American female swimmer became the first woman to swim across the English Channel. Upon returning home, she received a very large ticker-tape parade in New York City.
    Gertrude Ederle

2. This man, nicknamed "The Greatest," "The Champ," and "Louisville Lip," was one of the best heavyweight boxers of all time. He changed his birth name when he was a young man after he converted to Islam.
    Mohammed Ali

3. This runner won gold medals in both the decathlon and the pentathlon. He also excelled in many other sports, including football, baseball, and basketball. Being of mixed Native American and white ancestry, he struggled with racism throughout his sports career.
    Jim Thorpe

4. This great swimmer won an unprecedented seven events—all that he entered—in the 1972 summer Olympics in Germany.
    Mark Spitz

5. Perhaps the most famous baseball player of all time, this New York Yankee "Sultan of Swat" held the home run record of 60 in a season, until Roger Maris broke it in the early 1960s. He changed the game of baseball with his power and his personality.
    Babe Ruth

6. In 1947, this Brooklyn Dodger great became the first black major league baseball player in modern times. Inducted into the Hall of Fame in 1962, he was a member of six World Series winning teams and also won many other awards.
    Jackie Robinson

7. This man, one of the greatest golfers of all time, was nicknamed "The King." He won seven major championships between 1958 and 1964 and continued to play professionally until 2004.
    Arnold Palmer

8. This 7'1" basketball player was nicknamed " . . . the Stilt." He is the only player to average more than 50 points per game in a season and also the only one to score a whopping 100 points in a single game!
    Wilt Chamberlin

9. This female swimmer wrote an autobiography named *The Million Dollar Mermaid*. She went on from swimming to become a very successful movie star of the 1940s and '50s.
    Esther Williams

10. This world famous bike rider won an unprecedented seven consecutive Tour de France road races from 1999 to 2005. After courageously beating cancer, he began a foundation to fight the disease. His yellow "Live Strong" rubber bracelets have become popular throughout the world and have raised many millions of dollars to support his foundation.
    Lance Armstrong

11. This child prodigy began playing golf at age 2 and by age 8 was winning tournaments. In 2006, he was the highest paid athlete, winning $100 million in tournaments and endorsements! He has been the PGA Player of the Year eight times.
    Tiger Woods

12. This football great spent most of his years as quarterback for the New York Jets, beginning in 1965. His antics, both on and off the field, were legendary. He appeared in many advertisements and was especially known for Remington electric shaver ads. His nickname is "Broadway . . ."
    Joe Namath

Reprinted from *Strengthen Your Mind, Volume Two* by Einberger & Sellick.
© 2008 by Health Professions Press, Inc.

Exercise Puzzle

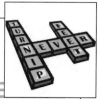

Below is the word *exercise* listed twice. Create a new word using a combination of the two words together. The new word can be any length, as long as it uses the same letter from both columns.

Example:

E n E rgy

E   E

X   X

E   E

R   R

C   C

I   I

S   S

E   E

Strategies for Memory Improvement

Strategies for Memory Improvement
FACILITATOR OVERVIEW

Many books have been written on how to improve memory, including strategies to prevent memory loss and techniques to remember bits of information. This lesson will teach participants the most effective and easy strategies to help keep their memory sharp as well as how to incorporate the strategies into everyday life. These strategies should give participants plenty of material to practice with. They are time-tested tips that can help a person to remember any type of information and can be used anytime or anywhere.

PAYING ATTENTION

It may sound simple, but paying attention is at the top of the list when it comes to strategies for improving memory. Many memory complaints can actually be traced to lack of focus or too much multitasking, both of which can inhibit the ability to remember. For example, if you are making a doctor's appointment on the phone and you are also making dinner with the television on in the background, your brain is focusing on three different tasks rather than just one. If you give your brain the maximum opportunity to absorb information, you will be more likely to remember it. Make it your *intention to pay attention!*

VISUALIZATION

Visualization involves taking a picture of something in your mind's eye and using that image to help remember the item. According to the book *Memory Fitness: A Guide for Successful Aging*, creating a visual image of an item that you want to remember will make it easier to remember the item by forcing you to make the information more specific or particular and less arbitrary (Einstein and McDaniel, 2003). For example, if you want to remember the name of a new coworker (Jane), you could visualize her standing on her desk jumping up and down. Although it sounds silly, the more exaggerated or outlandish the visualization is, the more likely you will remember it.

CHUNKING

As was mentioned as part of the class on Memory and Aging, short-term memory can hold only about five to nine items. Chunking is a strategy that breaks large pieces of information into smaller chunks so that they are easier to hold in short-term memory. For example, if you are going to the grocery store and have a list of 12 items that you need to buy, break down the list into four groups of three items that are somehow associated with each other. A list of milk, croutons, dog food, rice, lunch meat, crackers, cheese, chicken, eggs, laundry soap, hot dogs, and shampoo could be broken down into the following groups:

Dairy—milk, eggs, cheese

Starch—rice, crackers, croutons

Meat—chicken, hot dogs, lunch meat

Household items—dog food, laundry soap, shampoo

MNEMONICS

Mnemonics are phrases that help you to remember lists or specific information. In elementary school, many people learned the mnemonic Roy G. Biv to remember the colors of the rainbow (red, orange, yellow, green, blue, indigo, violet), or All Cows Eat Grass to remember music notes. As with association, the more silly or creative the mnemonic, the more likely you will be successful at remembering the information. A mnemonic is very similar to an acronym, which is another good memory strategy. Both involve remembering information by using the first letter of a word to make up a word or sentence.

ASSOCIATION

Association involves connecting an item that you are trying to remember with something that you already know. One of the best examples of the use of association is when trying to remember a person's name. If you meet someone named Tom, think of another person you know (real or fictional) and "assign" his or her name to the person you just met. If you have a cousin named Tom, think of him, or if you don't know anyone named Tom, use Tom Hanks or another well-known individual with the name of Tom.

REPETITION

There is no doubt that continuously repeating information to yourself can help you remember. According to Nelson (2005), repetition can help you encode information by forcing you to pay attention to the information. You are more likely to remember a person's name if you repeat it immediately after hearing it the first time. The same applies for other information you are trying to remember. For example, if you are given a phone number and need to remember it for a few seconds or minutes before you have the chance to write it down or to dial the number, you can repeat it over and over. Or, if you want to remember the date that you are going on vacation, you can repeat it to yourself until you have the chance to write it down on a calendar or until the date sticks in your memory.

CREATING A STORY

Creating a story to link bits of information together is a proven way to help remember. For example, if you have three errands to run—get the car oil changed, pick up dry cleaning, and mail a letter—your story could go like this: You were on your way to mail a letter when you slipped on some oil and now need to drop off your clothes at the dry cleaners. Again, the more silly the story the better!

VISUAL REMINDERS

A visual reminder involves physically moving an item so that it is out of place and more likely to catch your eye. The key to this strategy is to make the item stand out, not so as to confuse you, but rather to trigger your memory. For example, if you are cooking something on the stove and you need to remember to check on it in 15 minutes, you could place an empty sauce pan on top of the television. Pans are usually kept in the kitchen, so the sauce pan will catch your eye and remind you to check on your food. Or, if you need to remember to water the flowers, place a watering can in front of a door or at the foot of your bed—anywhere you are more likely to notice it.

USING THE ALPHABET

A word or name that is "stuck" in your memory can sometimes be retrieved by saying each letter of the alphabet. When you reach the letter that the word you are trying to think of begins with, saying the letter will often stimulate your memory and enable you to recall the word. You can say the alphabet to yourself or out loud. For example, if you are trying to think of the name Nancy, when you get to the letter N your brain may be triggered to recall the name.

Strategies for Memory Improvement
FACILITATOR INSTRUCTIONS

1. WELCOME AND INTRODUCTION (10 MINUTES)

To do before class:

- Read and familiarize yourself with the Strategies for Memory Improvement Overview.
- Write the following quote on a board or flip chart.

> "Nothing fixes a thing so intensely in the memory as the wish to forget it."
> (Michel de Montaigne, French Renaissance writer)

- Familiarize yourself with and make appropriate copies of the warm-up activity, quiz, handout, practice activities, and homework.

Greet the participants and make introductions, if necessary. Explain that this lesson will teach them several strategies that can help to improve their memory. The strategies are easily learned and can help in remembering such things as names, lists, places, and so forth. Not all of the strategies will work well for everyone. Participants will learn and practice each strategy and choose which ones best help them.

Discuss the quote and ask participants for their interpretations. What makes something important enough to remember? Has anyone ever forgotten an important date, such as a birthday or anniversary?

2. WARM-UP ACTIVITY (10 MINUTES)

Pass out the worksheet *How Do You Remember?* and explain that many of us already have our own "bag of tricks" for remembering information. Encourage participants to list some of the ways they would try to remember the information on the page. After about 5 minutes, ask participants to share their ideas. They will most likely have some ideas that are examples of the strategies that will be discussed in class. Thank them for sharing and explain that they will learn more about strategies to improve memory during class.

3. MEMORY STRATEGIES QUIZ (15 MINUTES)

Pass out the Memory Strategies Quiz and explain that the true or false statements are related to memory strategies that will be discussed in class. After everyone has finished marking true or false, review the answers to each statement. Ask how participants did on the quiz and if anyone was surprised by some of the answers.

4. EXPLANATION AND DISCUSSION OF STRATEGIES FOR MEMORY IMPROVEMENT (15 MINUTES)

List the nine memory-improvement strategies from the Facilitator Overview on a board or flip chart and explain each. Tell participants that these strategies can help them to recall information more readily and are easily learned if practiced regularly. Explain that they will have the opportunity to familiarize themselves with some of the strategies in a few minutes. After the discussion, distribute the *Memory Strategies* handout and encourage participants to refer to it in the coming weeks.

5. PRACTICE ACTIVITIES (30 MINUTES)

Explain to participants that they are going to practice as a group a couple of strategies for remembering names. Ask each participant to get up and find someone in the class who they do not know. Ask them to introduce themselves to the person and to spend a few minutes talking with and getting to know each other. Then ask participants to try and remember the person's name by associating him or her with someone or something else. Ask participants to remember the association for a few minutes while they go on next to practice the technique of visualization. Ask them to visualize their new friend's name in the following two ways:

- Visualize the person's name in lights above the person's head
- Visualize the person's name written on a nametag on his or her shirt.

After about a minute, explain that these visualization techniques are two of the easiest ways to remember a name. Then ask participants to share what or whom they associated their new friend's name with.

Pass out the worksheet *Practicing Memory-Improvement Strategies* and explain that participants will have the opportunity to practice a few of the different strategies that they learned earlier. (Note: Depending on the number of participants, you may want to break up the group into three or four smaller groups of about five participants and let them work together.) After most have finished, ask participants to share some of their answers. Note that answers will vary with this activity. Possible answers for number 3B (Mnemonics) may include the following:

- All Cool Cows Eat Peas
- Perfect Cats Are Easy Cats
- C-CAPE

6. REVIEW AND CLOSING (5 MINUTES)

Quickly go over the strategies learned in class and encourage participants to choose one or two of them to practice this week. Remind everyone that one of the best and easiest ways to remember most efficiently is to really *pay attention* to what it is that they want to remember. Have everyone repeat, "Make it your intention to pay attention!"

7. HOMEWORK (5 MINUTES)

Pass out the homework sheets, explain what should be done for each, and encourage participants to fill them out during the week. Remind them that homework should be fun and suggest that they enlist the help of family and friends, if they can.

- *Using Memory Strategies in Everyday Life*
- *Places and Things Named for People*
- Practice, practice, practice your memory enhancement strategies!

Strategies for Memory Improvement
CLASS AGENDA

1. Welcome and Introduction
2. Warm-Up Activity
   - *How Do You Remember?*
3. Memory Strategies Quiz
4. Overview of Strategies to Improve Memory
   - Paying attention
   - Visualization
   - Chunking
   - Mnemonics
   - Association
   - Repetition
   - Using Stories
   - Visual Reminders
   - Using the Alphabet
5. Practice Activities
   - Remembering Names (Group Activity)
   - *Practicing Memory-Improvement Strategies*
6. Review and Closing
7. Homework
   - *Using Memory Strategies in Everyday Life*
   - *Places and Things Named for People*
   - Practice, practice, practice your memory enhancement strategies!

Strengthen Your Mind Program: A Course for Memory Enhancement by Einberger & Sellick.
© 2010 by Health Professions Press, Inc.

How Do You Remember?

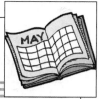

Many of us have memory "tricks" that we use to help us remember bits of information. Look at the items below and list a way that you would try to remember the information.

1. A list of items that you need from the grocery store.

2. The name of someone you've met for the first time.

3. The time a movie is showing.

4. A doctor's appointment.

5. Important information that you need to pass on to a friend.

Memory Strategies Quiz

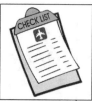

Write *T* for *true* or *F* for *false* on the line before each statement.

_____ 1.   Writing things down is a crutch that can actually weaken memory.

_____ 2.   Repeating information over and over can confuse your brain and make it less likely that you will remember it.

_____ 3.   As you get older it becomes more difficult to learn new memory strategies.

_____ 4.   Bizarre or silly bits of information are easier to remember.

_____ 5.   Many memory issues are due to not paying attention or being distracted.

_____ 6.   As you grow older it becomes more difficult to remember names.

_____ 7.   Using visualization distracts your brain from absorbing and remembering information.

_____ 8.   Mnemonics are useful tools for young children to remember information for school, not for older adults trying to remember information for daily life.

_____ 9.   Chunking is only useful for trying to remember sequences of numbers.

_____ 10. If practiced regularly, memory improvement strategies can help you to recall information more efficiently.

Strengthen Your Mind Program: A Course for Memory Enhancement by Einberger & Sellick.

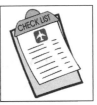

F   1. **Writing things down is a crutch that can actually weaken memory.**
Writing things down is a tool that when used as necessary can help to improve memory by keeping stress levels down.

F   2. **Repeating information over and over can confuse your brain and make it less likely that you will remember it.**
Repeating things over and over is a well-known memory strategy that forces your brain to pay attention to information.

F   3. **As you get older it becomes more difficult to learn new memory strategies.**
Memory improvement strategies can be learned at any age. As you get older, however, you may have to practice them more than when you were younger.

T   4. **Bizarre or silly bits of information are easier to remember.**
When using memory strategies, the more outlandish or creative the better.

T   5. **Many memory issues are due to not paying attention or being distracted.**
Not giving 100 percent of your attention to what you are trying to remember is a common cause of memory loss.

F   6. **As you grow older it becomes more difficult to remember names.**
Although it may take you longer to recall names, with normal aging you should not have more difficulty remembering them.

F   7. **Using visualization distracts your brain from absorbing and remembering information.**
Visualization is a powerful memory tool that can be used to remember almost any type of information.

F   8. **Mnemonics are useful tools for young children to remember information for school, not for older adults trying to remember information for daily life.**
Mnemonics can be used at any age and can be helpful for remembering lists and other sequential types of information.

F   9. **Chunking is only useful for trying to remember sequences of numbers.**
Chunking can be used to remember a variety of things, such as a grocery list.

T 10. **If practiced regularly, memory improvement strategies can help you to recall information more efficiently.**
Just like learning a new language, using memory strategies takes practice. The strategies you will learn about as part of this lesson are proven techniques that can help to improve your memory.

Strengthen Your Mind Program: A Course for Memory Enhancement by Einberger & Sellick.
© 2010 by Health Professions Press, Inc.

Memory Strategies

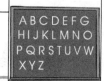

Paying Attention. Difficulty remembering can often be related to problems with focus. Pay attention to what you are doing and consciously focus on the fact that you are trying to remember something. Make it your *intention to pay attention!*

Visualization. If you are trying to remember something or someone, visualize the person or item with your mind's eye.

Chunking. Break down lists of information into manageable chunks of no more than three or four items.

Mnemonics. Create phrases that help you remember lists or specific information (e.g., Roy G. Biv or All Cows Eat Grass).

Association. Associate the item that you are trying to remember with something that will help you remember it. The more exaggerated or silly, the better!

Repetition. Repeating information over and over can help you to remember it. This technique, however, will only work if you are paying attention to what you are doing. Focus, focus, focus!

Creating a Story. Make up a story linking together all of the components of the information you are trying to remember.

Visual Reminders. Place an item in an unusual place to trigger your memory to recall something (e.g., a sauce pan on top of the television to remember to turn off the stove).

Using the Alphabet. Saying each letter of the alphabet can help you to recall a word or name.

Strengthen Your Mind Program: A Course for Memory Enhancement by Einberger & Sellick.

Practicing Memory-Improvement Strategies

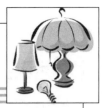

1. *Chunking.* Break down the following list of items into smaller "chunks."
    rose, Paris, soup, panda, grass, dog, kangaroo, navy beans, Cincinnati, Cypress, cupcakes, San Francisco, oak

2. *Visual Reminders.* What visual reminders would you use to remember the following items?

    A. Change a light bulb

    B. Take medication

    C. Call your cousin

    D. Take out a steak from the freezer

3. *Mnemonics.*

    A. What are some mnemonics that you used in school or when you were younger?

    B. Make up a mnemonic for the following list: eggs, chili, apples, cheese, pasta.

Using Memory Strategies in Everyday Life

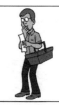

1. Choose at least one new memory strategy that you will try this week.

2. Which one did you choose and why?

3. What steps will you take to practice this strategy?

4. Did this strategy work for you? Why or why not?

Strengthen Your Mind Program: A Course for Memory Enhancement by Einberger & Sellick.

Places and Things Named for People

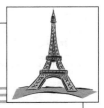

Not only do people name products after other people, but places and things are often namesakes as well. Some of the most noted tourist destinations in the world have been named for people, including our own continent. Match the description on the left to the answer on the right.

___ 1. Many contend that these two continents were named after Italian explorer Amerigo Vespucci, who believed that the continents were a previously undiscovered world.

___ 2. This Chicago baseball park is named after its owner, the same person who owns one of the most famous chewing gum companies in the world.

___ 3. This famous French landmark, named after its designer, stands 990 feet tall and was built for the 1889 International Exposition.

___ 4. This Los Angeles destination, originally called Mann's Chinese Theater, is the home of nearly 200 celebrity handprints, footprints, and autographs.

___ 5. This famous comet that was last seen in 1986 is visible every 75 to 76 years and was named after an English astronomer.

___ 6. This performing arts center in Washington, DC, was designated as a memorial to a famous president who was assassinated in 1963.

___ 7. This theme park is known for being the "Happiest Place on Earth" and is named after its creator, a legend in animation.

___ 8. This nationwide financial services company has over 6,000 branches and is named after the two men who created it in 1852.

___ 9. As one of the largest auto companies in the United States, this company was named after its founder and is over 100 years old.

___ 10. Over ten towers and plazas throughout the world are named after this real estate mogul and entertainer, one of the richest men in the United States.

___ 11. This item, popular with young children, was named after Theodore Roosevelt.

___ 12. Named after its creator, this line of foot care products includes shoes, inserts, lotions, and other foot-pampering items.

___ 13. Located in Vatican City, this site is named after one of the 12 apostles of Jesus.

___ 14. This Polish-born woman created a beauty empire and created a cosmetics business named after herself.

a. Wells Fargo

b. Eiffel Tower

c. Helena Rubenstein

d. Halley's Comet

e. Donald Trump

f. Dr. Scholl's

g. Grauman's Chinese Theatre

h. North and South America

i. St. Peter's Basilica

j. Disneyland

k. Ford Motor Company

l. The Kennedy Center

m. Teddy Bear

n. Wrigley Field

Places and Things Named for People

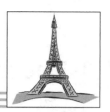

1. Many contend that these two continents were named after Italian explorer Amerigo Vespucci, who believed that the continents were a previously undiscovered world.

    h. North and South America

2. This Chicago baseball park is named after its owner, the same person who owns one of the most famous chewing gum companies in the world.

    n. Wrigley Field

3. This famous French landmark, named after its designer, stands 990 feet tall and was built for the 1889 International Exposition.

    b. Eiffel Tower

4. This Los Angeles destination, originally called Mann's Chinese Theater, is the home of nearly 200 celebrity handprints, footprints, and autographs.

    g. Grauman's Chinese Theatre

5. This famous comet that was last seen in 1986 is visible every 75 to 76 years and was named after an English astronomer.

    d. Halley's Comet

6. This performing arts center in Washington, DC, was designated as a memorial to a famous president who was assassinated in 1963.

    l. The Kennedy Center

7. This theme park is known for being the "Happiest Place on Earth" and is named after its creator, a legend in animation.

    j. Disneyland

8. This nationwide financial services company has over 6,000 branches and is named after the two men who created it in 1852.

    a. Wells Fargo

9. As one of the largest auto companies in the United States, this company was named after its founder and is over 100 years old.

    k. Ford Motor Company

10. Over ten towers and plazas throughout the world are named after this real estate mogul and entertainer, one of the richest men in the United States.

    e. Donald Trump

11. This item, popular with young children, was named after Theodore Roosevelt.

    m. Teddy Bear

12. Named after its creator, this line of foot care products includes shoes, inserts, lotions, and other foot-pampering items.

    f. Dr. Scholl's

13. Located in Vatican City, this site is named after one of the 12 apostles of Jesus.

    i. St. Peter's Basilica

14. This Polish-born woman created a beauty empire and created a cosmetics business named after herself.

    c. Helena Rubenstein

Reprinted from *Strengthen Your Mind, Volume Two* by Einberger & Sellick.
© 2008 by Health Professions Press, Inc.

Brain Dominance

Brain Dominance
FACILITATOR OVERVIEW

For the most part, people use one side of their brain more often and more efficiently than the other in thinking and learning. The truth is, however, that people use both sides of their brain and that most do so in a fairly unbalanced way. This lesson will explain what it means to be left-brained or right-brained as well as the importance of using the whole brain to enhance memory.

RIGHT BRAIN VERSUS LEFT BRAIN

The right and left brains, or hemispheres, control the opposite side of the body (i.e., the right brain controls the left side of the body, and the left brain controls the right side of the body). Those who more often use the right side of their body are primarily left-brained and those who more often use the left side of their body are generally right-brained. A person does, of course, have only one brain, and this unique organ is made up of two halves that are connected by a mass of nerves.

In the late 1960s and early 1970s, Roger W. Sperry, a Nobel prize winner from the United States, studied the relationship between the brain's right and left hemispheres and discovered that the human brain has two different ways of thinking. The right side of the brain is visual and intuitive and looks at the whole rather than the individual parts. The left side of the brain is verbal and analytical and looks first at each individual part in sequence and then puts the parts together to make a whole.

Many years after Roger Sperry's findings, Ned Herrmann, former Manager of Management Education at General Electric's Management Development Institute, developed a brain-dominance instrument to assess the primary way in which a person uses his or her brain. His research in brain-dominance theory found that people in various professions tend to be either primarily right-brained or left-brained, depending on the type of work they do within that profession. For example, administrative assistants are generally left-brained because they need to do their work in a sequential, organized, and timely manner.

USING THE WHOLE BRAIN

What may be most important in discussing brain dominance and its relationship to memory is to know that people use different sides of their brains to process different kinds of information. People prefer, for the most part, to be taught and to learn using their strengths, and often rely more heavily on the dominant side of their brain.

Although most of us prefer to use learning strategies that are associated with either the right or left side, the two sides of the brain do, in fact, work together in our daily lives. Also, it is possible to strengthen the nondominant side of the brain. Not only is it possible, it is extremely valuable in learning ways to enhance memory. The more efficiently *both* sides of the brain are used, the more "brain power" a person has to help with memory!

In teaching this class as well as all of the others, it is important to keep in mind that we as teachers tend to use teaching techniques associated with our specific brain dominance. Left-brained teachers, therefore, may be more verbal and analytical in their teaching, whereas right-brained teachers may use more visuals, group work, and music. To successfully teach both left- and right-brained learners, we, as teachers or facilitators, need to practice using the nondominant side of our brain. Not only will this be beneficial for participants, it will also help us to use our whole brain more efficiently.

The handout *What Does It Mean to Be Left-brained or Right-brained?* summarizes the characteristics generally associated with and the differences between the two sides of the brain and will be helpful in teaching yourself as well as participants how to effectively use the whole brain to enhance memory.

Brain Dominance
FACILITATOR INSTRUCTIONS

1. WELCOME AND INTRODUCTION (10 MINUTES)

To do before class:

- Read and familiarize yourself with the Brain Dominance Overview as well as the handout *What Does It Mean to Be Left-brained or Right-brained?*

- Write the following quotes on a board or flip chart.

> "Begin challenging your own assumptions. Your assumptions are your windows on the world. Scrub them off every once in a while, or the light won't come in."
> (Alan Alda, actor)

> "Think left and think right and think low and think high. Oh, the thinks you can think up if only you try!" (from *Oh, the Thinks You Can Think!*, Theodor Geisel [Dr. Seuss], author and illustrator)

> "You can't depend on your eyes when your imagination is out of focus."
> (Mark Twain, author and humorist)

- Familiarize yourself with and make appropriate copies of the warm-up activity, quiz, practice activities, and homework.

Greet the participants and make introductions, if necessary. Ask them whether they believe they are right-brained or left-brained, without giving much of an explanation. Let them know that by the end of the class they will have a good idea as to which side of their brain they use the majority of the time.

The three quotes all relate to brain dominance. Use one, two, or all of them for discussion, asking participants for their interpretations.

2. WARM-UP ACTIVITY (10 MINUTES) (GROUP ACTIVITY)

Put a large paper bag (the type you get at the grocery store) on a table or someplace where everyone can see it. Ask participants to list five things that the bag could be used for, besides putting groceries into. Encourage them to think outside the box. Give them 5 minutes to brainstorm before you ask for answers. Explain to them that this is an activity that uses the right side of the brain, as they have to use their imagination in new, creative ways.

Possible answers may include to:

Use as a rain hat

Wrap a package

Make book covers

Use as stationary to write a letter

Use as a fire starter

Roll up and swat flies

Decorate and use as a Halloween costume, mask, or bag for a young child

Cover a plant in the winter

Use as protection over pictures when painting.

3. QUIZ (10 MINUTES)

Ask participants to complete the *Brain Dominance Questionnaire* and then add up their totals. Ask for a show of hands as to how many people are left-brained. Right-brained? Do they agree with the assessment? They may have a better idea after the explanation and review of the handout *What Does It Mean to Be Left-brained or Right-brained?*

4. EXPLANATION AND DISCUSSION OF BRAIN DOMINANCE AND HOW IT AFFECTS MEMORY (20 MINUTES)

Explain to participants that this lesson identifies the characteristics of the left and right sides of the brain, helps them to assess which side they use the most, and provides tips for using the nondominant side of the brain more frequently and efficiently.

After summarizing the overview, briefly discuss the meaning of brain dominance and its history. Be sure to point out that those who are left-brained are not more intelligent than those who are right-brained or vice versa. We simply process information differently and have different modes of thinking.

Next, distribute the handout *What Does It Mean to Be Left-brained or Right-brained?* Review each list and ask for comments or questions from participants. Reiterate that in order to use our brains more effectively, we need to go beyond simply knowing which side of our brain we use most. We also need to learn ways to use the nondominant side of our brain and incorporate both sides into our thinking in order to make us more "whole-brained."

5. PRACTICE ACTIVITIES (30 MINUTES)

Pass out *Tips for Using Your Whole Brain*. Review the list with the class and ask for additional suggestions. Note how important it is to use both sides of the brain. Encourage participants to use these tips to help themselves to become more whole-brained.

After the discussion, let participants know that they will next have the opportunity to work on two activities. One will force them to use the nondominant side of their brain, and the other will teach them to use both sides of their brain at the same time.

First, pass out the activity *Writing with Your Nondominant Hand*. Ask participants to rewrite this paragraph using whichever hand they don't ordinarily use to write. This will force them to use the opposite (nondominant) side of their brain.

Next, if time permits, divide the participants into two groups and ask them to brainstorm (typically a right-brain activity) and then list (typically a left-brain activity) who they think are the top five U.S. presidents in order of the time periods they served (typically a left-brain activity).

6.   REVIEW AND CLOSING (5 MINUTES)

Thank the group for their participation. Quickly review the main points of what it means to be left- or right-brained. Note how important it is that we use both sides of the brain as fully as possible in order to enhance memory. Explain that the goal is not for participants to stop using the dominant side of their brain, but rather for them to use their nondominant side more than they currently do. Encourage participants to be more whole-brained in the future.

7.   HOMEWORK (5 MINUTES)

Pass out the homework sheets, explain what should be done for each, and emphasize the importance of completing the assignments. Tell participants that the worksheets are great ways to enhance their memory by using their whole brain.

- *Using the Opposite (Nondominant) Side of Your Brain*

- *Composers*

- Pay attention to which side of your body you use the most, and practice using the other side often!

Brain Dominance
CLASS AGENDA

1. Welcome and Introduction
2. Warm-Up Activity
   - A Grocery Bag! (Group Activity)
3. *Brain Dominance Questionnaire*
4. *What Does It Mean to Be Left-brained or Right-brained?*
5. Practice Activities
   - *Tips for Using Your Whole Brain*
   - *Writing with Your Nondominant Hand*
   - Brainstorming (Top Five U.S. Presidents) (Group Activity)
6. Review and Closing
7. Homework
   - *Using the Opposite (Nondominant) Side of Your Brain*
   - *Composers*
   - Pay attention to which side of your body you use the most and practice using the other side often!

Brain Dominance Questionnaire

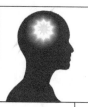

Choose the statement that is most true for you the majority of the time.

1. I learn best by
    A. Using details and specific facts.
    B. Looking at the whole picture first to gain an overview.

2. I remember people best by
    A. Their names.
    B. Their faces.

3. When I cross my arms
    A. My right arm is on top.
    B. My left arm is on top.

4. When I have to make a difficult decision, I'm more than likely to choose
    A. What I *know* is right.
    B. What I *think* is right.

5. When I need to solve a problem
    A. I use logic to look for the answer.
    B. I go with my "gut instinct."

6. When listening to someone speak, I gain greater knowledge of what they are saying by
    A. Listening to what they say.
    B. Observing their body language.

7. When solving problems
    A. I work on one at a time.
    B. I work on many at the same time.

8. When I explain directions to others
    A. I primarily use words.
    B. I use many gestures.

9. I remember things best
    A. With words.
    B. With pictures, diagrams, and illustrations.

10. When I cross my legs
    A. My right leg is on top.
    B. My left leg in on top.

Strengthen Your Mind Program: A Course for Memory Enhancement by Einberger & Sellick.
© 2010 by Health Professions Press, Inc.

11. When I'm assembling something, I'm likely to
    A. Gather the necessary tools first and then follow the directions step by step.
    B. Jump right in without studying the directions first.

12. When I have an appointment
    A. It is always my priority to arrive on time.
    B. It is hard to arrive on time when I'm in the middle of something else.

13. Regarding creativity
    A. I do not consider myself creative.
    B. I consider myself fairly creative in one area or another or maybe many areas.

14. It is easier to wink with my
    A. Right eye closed.
    B. Left eye closed.

15. Before I begin a discussion about a project
    A. I like to get all of the facts.
    B. I like to jump right in and start brainstorming with others.

16. During lectures
    A. I pay close attention to what the speaker is saying.
    B. I often doodle.

17. When I'm working
    A. I like my day to be well planned.
    B. I am always open to new possibilities and opportunities for change.

18. Regarding risks
    A. I usually do not like to take them and can have fun without them.
    B. I enjoy taking them and feel I need some risks in my life.

19. When you bring your hands together and interlock your fingers, which thumb is on top?
    A. Right.
    B. Left.

20. Others tell me that
    A. I am well organized.
    B. They don't quite understand how I organize things or how I find things.

21. In my life, I like
    A. Things structured and well planned.
    B. A variety of things to do and places to go.

22. People would say that
    A   I am a stable person and am consistent in my actions.
    B. I am a flexible person and often unpredictable.

SCORING:

Number of As _____

Number of Bs _____

As generally represent left-brained characteristics and Bs generally represent those of the right brain. In which category did you score higher? Most of us are predominantly left-brained or right-brained, but we should all strive to use both sides of our brain somewhat equally in order to maximize our memory. How could you do this?

Strengthen Your Mind Program: A Course for Memory Enhancement by Einberger & Sellick.

What Does It Mean to Be Left-brained or Right-brained?

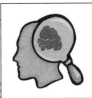

If you are predominantly *left-brained*, most of these characteristics probably fit you:

You are verbal.
You are analytical and detail oriented.
You are logical.
You are sequential (you process information in sequence).
You use words to remember things.
You remember names better than faces.
You read all of the information and then make a logical deduction.
You work step by step, focusing on details.
You like to make lists and plans.
You are good at keeping track of time.
You enjoy observing.
You plan ahead.
You are likely to read an instruction manual.
You read for details and facts.
You like to do things independently of others.
You listen to *what* is being said.
You rarely use gestures in conversation.
You tend to believe that you're not creative, although this isn't necessarily true.

If you are predominately *right-brained*, most of these characteristics probably fit you:

You learn well nonverbally.
You often make decisions based on intuition and are led by your feelings.
You are often unpredictable and spontaneous.
You like to move while thinking.
You daydream and use your imagination frequently.
Your organization seems to be lacking at times.
You like to know why you're doing something or why rules exist.
You do not have a good sense of time.
You enjoy touching and feeling objects to learn more about them.
You often talk with your hands.
You listen to *how* something is being said.
You like to look at the whole first and then check out the details. You're a "big-picture" person.
You remember faces better than names.
You are often thought to be philosophical in your thinking.
You become restless during long verbal explanations and are anxious to "get on with it."
You are unlikely to read an instruction manual before assembling an item.
You use pictures to remember things, whether in your mind or on paper.

Tips for Using Your Whole Brain

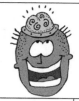

In order to have a more balanced brain, try to use the nondominant side of your brain more frequently. Read through the tips below and pick at least one that you will use to help make your brain more balanced, or more "whole-brained"!

If you are predominantly left-brained:
- Exercise your creativity (paint, sing, cook, write).
- Think "outside the box" more often rather than analytically.
- Think about things as a whole and then check out the details.
- Use your imagination.
- Be spontaneous at times.
- Ask "why?" more often.
- Use color-coding to help you organize.
- Do activities that are hands-on.
- Take mental pictures of things you want to remember.
- Practice using your nondominant hand.
- Cross your hands, arms, and legs in the opposite direction of how you usually cross them.
- Brainstorm goals for yourself.
- Brainstorm with others.
- Use visualization and illustrations to help you remember.
- Take risks.

If you are predominantly right-brained:
- Practice math problems and calculations.
- Set up rules, guidelines, or schedules for yourself.
- Practice listening and observing more closely.
- Play games that involve logic or deduction.
- Use lists, a calendar, or a date book to become better organized.
- Practice using your nondominant hand.
- Cross your hands, arms, and legs in the opposite direction of how you usually cross them.
- Set goals for yourself with sequential steps to achieve each.
- Work on projects independently of others at times.
- Follow written directions.
- Pay attention to details.
- Use words to help you remember.

Writing with Your Nondominant Hand

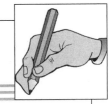

Using your nondominant hand, copy the short paragraph below.

I woke up this morning to a wonderfully sunny day. Birds were chirping, the coffee was brewing, music was playing, and all my senses were alive. It was the beginning of what would be a great day!

Strengthen Your Mind Program: A Course for Memory Enhancement by Einberger & Sellick.

Using the Opposite (Nondominant) Side of Your Brain

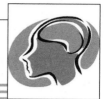

List five ways in which you will strive to use the nondominant side of your brain in the coming week. Use ideas that have been discussed in class and/or tips from the list *Tips for Using Your Whole Brain*.

1.

2.

3.

4.

5.

How will you remember to do these?

Were you successful? If so, can you continue to use the nondominant side of your brain in other ways? If you were not successful, what could you do to become more successful?

Composers

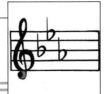

The following songs were all written by famous composers. Use your left brain and your right brain to identify each composer. Many are used more than once. The answers are listed (out of order) at the bottom of the page.

1. "Beautiful Dreamer"

2. "Easter Parade"

3. "Don't Fence Me In"

4. "You're a Grand Old Flag"

5. "This Land Is Your Land"

6. "Oh, Susannah"

7. "Oh, What a Beautiful Morning!"

8. "I Got Rhythm"

9. "God Bless America"

10. "Give My Regards to Broadway"

11. "Edelweiss"

13. "Back in the Saddle"

14. "Always"

15. "Aloha 'Oe"

16. "Hey, Good Lookin'"

17. "Yankee Doodle Dandy"

18. "White Christmas"

Irving Berlin   Rodgers and Hammerstein   George and Ira Gershwin
George M. Cohan   Julia Ward Howe   Gene Autry   Stephen Foster
Woody Guthrie   Queen Lili'uokalani   Hank Williams, Sr.   Cole Porter

Composers ANSWER SHEET

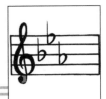

1.	"Beautiful Dreamer"	**Stephen Foster**
2.	"Easter Parade"	**Irving Berlin**
3.	"Don't Fence Me In"	**Cole Porter**
4.	"You're a Grand Old Flag"	**George M. Cohan**
5.	"This Land Is Your Land"	**Woody Guthrie**
6.	"Oh, Susannah"	**Stephen Foster**
7.	"Oh, What a Beautiful Morning!"	**Rodgers and Hammerstein**
8.	"I Got Rhythm"	**George and Ira Gershwin**
9.	"God Bless America"	**Irving Berlin**
10.	"Give My Regards to Broadway"	**George M. Cohan**
11.	"Edelweiss"	**Rodgers and Hammerstein**
12.	"Battle Hymn of the Republic"	**Julia Ward Howe (and William Steffe)**
13.	"Back in the Saddle"	**Gene Autry (and Ray Whitley)**
14.	"Always"	**Irving Berlin**
15.	"Aloha 'Oe"	**Queen Lili'uokalani**
16.	"Hey, Good Lookin'"	**Hank Williams, Sr.**
17.	"Yankee Doodle Dandy"	**George M. Cohan**
18.	"White Christmas"	**Irving Berlin**

Strengthen Your Mind Program: A Course for Memory Enhancement by Einberger & Sellick.

The Five Senses

The Five Senses
FACILITATOR OVERVIEW

We all have five senses—sight, hearing, touch, taste, and smell. As we grow older some of our senses may not be as sharp as they once were, but for the most part we all can make adjustments to compensate for these changes. We can also learn to use all of our senses more fully.

We've all heard the expression "take time to smell the roses," but in our busy, everyday lives many of us don't do this. We don't stop and really smell the rose, touch it, and look at it. All too often we don't really think about all that our senses have to offer. Everything we know and learn comes to us through our senses. The more consciously we use all of our senses, the more information we collect and the easier that information is to recall. In other words, the more information we receive through a variety of paths, the more likely we are to remember the information. If we truly use all of our senses in combination with one another, we stand the greatest likelihood of being able to enhance our memories. This lesson focuses on encouraging participants to do just that.

The following is a short overview of each of the senses. For more scientific explanations, you may want to research each sense individually. What the authors have found to be most important is to identify for participants ways in which they can use each of the five senses in their everyday lives and to encourage them to use their senses in combination with one another. The tips and activities that are a part of this lesson will help participants to sharpen their senses.

As you encourage participants to use all of their senses more in everyday life, it is important that you set an example and use all of the five senses in teaching this lesson. Use visuals, have music or other sounds for participants to listen to, encourage them to touch (papers, fabrics, different writing utensils), bring in different aromas for them to smell and food to taste, and so forth. This lesson on senses can be done in one class, but can also be done more thoroughly in multiple classes.

SIGHT

Most of the information we take in is based on what we see. Experts estimate that as much as 90% of what we learn is through sight. Along with hearing, sight is what we most depend on to be able to lead our daily lives safely and efficiently. It is also the most complex of all of our senses, although it is not the strongest when it comes to memories. One problem with gaining information through our sense of sight is that often we look but we don't really see. We simply do not pay close enough attention to what we are seeing and, therefore, should not rely on sight alone to help us remember things.

Consider, for example, the following situation: You meet someone new and important at the grocery store and you really want to remember what she looks like so that you can tell your friend. Meanwhile, your cell phone rings with your husband letting you know that you need to buy milk. At the same time, you are checking your grocery list to see if milk is on it. A few minutes later you meet your friend and begin to tell her about the person you met. Much to your dismay, you don't remember many details. This is a classic example of not paying close attention. Your intention was to remember as much as you could about the person, but you were distracted by both your grocery shopping and your telephone call and simply did not lend enough attention to studying how the person looked.

A better approach would have been to ignore the telephone call and really concentrate on the new acquaintance. An even better approach would have been to use all of your senses to remember the person. What was she wearing? What color were her eyes, hair, and so forth? What was her hairstyle? How did she talk? If you touched her clothes or her skin, what do you think they would feel like? Smooth? Rough? Silky? Was she wearing a particular perfume? As mentioned earlier, the more senses we use in garnering information, the more likely we are going to be able to remember.

HEARING

As we age, many of us experience a decline in hearing. This can be very problematic to memory, so we need to pay closer attention and practice listening. Second only to sight, hearing is the sense that we use most. We take in 10% to 15% of information through what we hear.

One important factor in maximizing the sense of hearing is to minimize auditory distractions. Especially for those of us who rely heavily on the sense of hearing to take in new information, we need to focus on listening to one thing at a time. If you're having an important conversation with someone, you need to pay attention to that person and what is being said (e.g., turn off the television and the radio, unless it's simply nice background music without words). If you're having a telephone conversation, make sure no one is trying to talk to you at the same time, which would lessen your ability to concentrate and, therefore, to remember.

The combined senses of sight and hearing account for most of the information we take in. The other three senses of touch, taste, and smell don't get used nearly as often as they can, and account for only 5% to 10% of the information we learn. It is essential for this lesson that participants learn to use the senses of touch, taste, and smell much more often than they most likely do at present.

TOUCH

Whereas the senses of sight, hearing, taste, and smell are found in specific parts of the body, the sense of touch is found throughout the body. The skin contains a multitude of different receptors, or nerve endings, that sense things such as pain, temperature, and pressure. These receptors then activate sensors that carry information to the brain. The sense of touch tells us how the world "feels," informs us of impending danger, registers whether we are happy or sad, and lets us know if something is rough or smooth.

All too often in our everyday lives we are urged not to touch things. Don't walk here. Please don't touch. No standing allowed. Lovely to look at, delightful to hold, but if you should break it, consider it sold! Whereas babies use the sense of touch to garner so much information about the world around them, adults are often urged not to do so. It's no wonder that the sense of touch is so little used!

Think about all that we touch during the day—a pillow, water in the shower, a spoon at breakfast, a coffee cup, a pen, a keyboard, clothes, the grass under your feet, the telephone, the remote control, a friend or relative's shoulder or hand, food at the grocery store, and so forth. Because so much of what we touch comes to us subconsciously, we need to make a more concerted effort to really pay attention to what we touch, which will then allow information to become more firmly placed in our memories.

TASTE

Although taste is the weakest of the five senses, it is very important to memory. Things that we tasted in our childhood can, after 50 years, still evoke many memories. Think back to your mother's special recipe or to the first Thanksgiving meal you ever prepared. Chances are you will still remember some emotions associated with that time.

We have five basic tastes—sour, sweet, bitter, salty, and umami (the taste found in cooked meats, mushrooms, or monosodium glutamate [MSG]). Each of the five has at least one receptor on the tongue, which is covered with thousands of tiny taste buds. When we eat, our saliva helps to break down food, which causes the receptors on the tongue to send messages to the brain that tell us what flavors we are eating (salty, sweet, sour, a combination).

As we grow older we lose taste buds, and the sense of taste decreases. This is one of the reasons that older people often add a lot of sugar or salt to their foods, to create a stronger taste. In terms of health, however, a better choice is to add herbs and spices and/or to try incorporating ethnic foods into your diet (Chinese, Mexican, Italian).

Experts say that up to 90% of what we taste is actually through the sense of smell. Most of what we call *flavor* comes from the aromas that reach nerves at the back of the throat through the nasal passages. A good indicator of this is to eat a food with a strong flavor with your nose plugged. Chances are you will not be able to identify the flavor by taste alone.

When it comes to using the sense of taste more, as with the other senses, you need to really pay attention to what you eat. This will help you to better store tastes in your memory. Practice identifying new tastes, try new recipes, use a greater variety of seasonings, and really think about the taste of each bite.

SMELL

Inside the top part of the nose is a small patch of tissue that contains millions of nerve cells. Odor sensors lie on these nerve cells, and each of them recognizes several odors. Although the sense of smell decreases with age, most of us still have the ability to recognize thousands of different smells as we get older.

Smell reaches the brain faster than any of the other senses. It does so almost instantaneously. It is the only sense that connects directly to the part of the brain called the limbic system, which is involved in storing memories and processing emotions. This is the reason why most experts agree that the sense of smell triggers memories more than any of the other four senses. Just think of some of your favorite smells—freshly mowed grass, newly baked cookies, popcorn, your favorite rose, that new car smell. All of these smells can evoke a multitude of memories from the past, memories that can last forever.

In *The Remembrance of Things Past*, French-novelist Marcel Proust wrote of the power of smell. He described what happened to him after he drank a spoonful of tea in which had soaked a piece of madeleine, a type of French cake:

> No sooner had the warm liquid mixed with the crumbs touched my palate than a shudder ran through my whole body, and I stopped, intent upon the extraordinary thing that was happening to me. . . . An exquisite pleasure had invaded my senses . . . with no suggestion of its origin. . . . Suddenly the memory revealed itself. The taste was of a little piece of Madeleine which on Sunday mornings . . . my Aunt Leonie used to give me, dipping it first in her own cup of tea. . . . Immediately the old gray house on

the street, where her room was, rose up like a stage set . . . and the entire town, with its people and houses, gardens, church, and surroundings, taking shape and solidity, sprang into being from my cup of tea.

Just seeing the madeleine had not brought back these memories, Proust noted. He needed to taste and smell it. "When nothing else subsists from the past," he wrote, "after the people are dead, after the things are broken and scattered . . . the smell and taste of things remain poised a long time, like souls . . . bearing resiliently, on tiny and almost impalpable drops of their essence, the immense edifice of memory."

Proust's discovery in the early part of the 1900s is still discussed today. Many have found the same effects of smell on memory. We need to pay close attention to all of the smells we encounter in our everyday lives as a way of sharpening our sense of smell and thereby enhancing our memory. Take time to smell the roses, the cake in the oven, the coffee brewing, and the newly laundered sheets!

The Five Senses
FACILITATOR INSTRUCTIONS

1. WELCOME AND INTRODUCTION (10 MINUTES)

To do before class:

- Read and familiarize yourself with The Five Senses Overview.
- Write the following quotes on a board or flip chart.

> "I want all my senses engaged. Let me absorb the
> world's variety and uniqueness."
> (Maya Angelou, poet)

> "Not the senses I have but what I do with them is my kingdom."
> (Helen Keller, author)

> "For the sense of smell, almost more than any other, has the power to recall
> memories and it is a pity that you use it so little."
> (Rachel Carson, environmentalist)

- Familiarize yourself with and make appropriate copies of the warm-up activity, practice activities, and homework.

Welcome participants and make introductions, if necessary. Explain that they will learn the importance of using all five of their senses to enhance their memory. Ask participants to name the five senses. Discuss the quotes and ask participants for their interpretations. Note the optimism and zest for life expressed in each.

2. WARM-UP ACTIVITY (10 MINUTES)

Pass out the warm-up activity *A Peaceful Place*. Review with participants the instructions and ask if they have any questions. Give them about 5 minutes to complete the activity. Then ask for volunteers to share their peaceful places.

3. WHICH SENSES DO WE USE THE MOST? (GROUP ACTIVITY) (5 MINUTES)

Ask participants to guess which sense people use the most to gather information from the environment. Then ask them how often they think the other senses are used.

Tell participants that research shows that at least 75% to 85% of knowledge comes from what we see, 10% to 15% from what we hear, and the remaining percentage from what we smell, touch, and taste. Discuss the relevance of the percentages. For example, how might they use the four lesser-used senses more in the future rather than depending so much on the sense of sight?

4. EXPLANATION AND DISCUSSION OF THE FIVE SENSES AND HOW THEY AFFECT MEMORY (25 MINUTES)

Explain to participants the importance of using each of their senses to enhance memory. Review the five senses, including some of the characteristics of each one. Be sure to read and discuss Marcel Proust's experience of the power of smell. Next, distribute the handout *Tips and Activities for Sharpening Your Senses*. Review the tips with participants, and encourage them to suggest possible additions to the list.

5. PRACTICE ACTIVITIES (30 MINUTES)

Tell participants that they will next complete two activities that will draw on all of their senses. Pass out the worksheet *Musical Instruments*. Divide participants into groups and give each group 5 to 7 minutes to complete the activity, reminding them to use *all* of their senses. After the groups have finished, spend a short time comparing answers.

Next, pass out the worksheet *Morning Time*. With participants still divided into groups, ask them to brainstorm how each of the senses is used first thing in the morning. If participants need a little coaching to get started, possible answers may be:

- The smell of coffee brewing or bacon frying or the smell of soap from the shower.
- Looking at yourself in the mirror or looking in a cupboard for something to make for breakfast.
- The feel of covers before getting out of bed or of water running down your body in the shower.
- The sound of an alarm clock or of birds chirping outside.
- The taste of that first cup of coffee, juice, milk, or tea.

Give the groups 5 to 7 minutes and then spend a short time comparing answers.

6.   REVIEW AND CLOSING (5 MINUTES)

Thank the group for their participation. Review with participants the importance of using *all* senses to take in as much information as possible. Although most of us tend to favor one sense as a means to garner information, we can learn to use the other four more efficiently to maximize memory. Let everyone know that you hope the information learned in class will help them to do just that.

7.   HOMEWORK (5 MINUTES)

Pass out the homework sheets and explain what should be done for each. Stress the importance of completing the assignments as practice in using as many of the senses as possible in everything they do.

- *Grocery Store Scavenger Hunt*

- *Well-Known Advertisements*

- Practice using all of your senses! And, as we hear so often, take time to smell the roses!

The Five Senses
CLASS AGENDA

1. Welcome and Introduction
2. Warm-Up Activity
   - *A Peaceful Place*
3. Which Senses Do We Use the Most? (Group Activity)
4. Explanation and Discussion of the Five Senses and How They Affect Memory
   - *Tips and Activities for Sharpening Your Senses*
5. Practice Activities
   - *Musical Instruments*
   - *Morning Time*
6. Review and Closing
7. Homework
   - *Grocery Store Scavenger Hunt*
   - *Well-Known Advertisements*
   - Practice using all of your senses!

A Peaceful Place

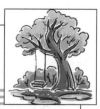

Close your eyes and imagine a very peaceful place outside where you could go and spend some time alone. Discover your surroundings. Look at all that's around you. Touch those things that are most appealing to you. Smell items that you believe may have a wonderful or memorable smell. Listen to all of the sounds. Imagine how some things would taste. Celebrate your senses! List two items you encountered on your journey in each of the following categories.

1. Listen

    A.

    B.

2. Look

    A.

    B.

3. Smell

    A.

    B.

4. Taste

    A.

    B.

5. Touch

    A.

    B.

Strengthen Your Mind Program: A Course for Memory Enhancement by Einberger & Sellick.

Tips and Activities for Sharpening Your Senses

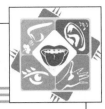

- Add spices and herbs to food instead of salt.
- If you smoke, quit now. Smoking adversely affects both your sense of smell and your sense of taste (not to mention your health).
- Take a walk and pay close attention to all that you see, hear, smell, and touch.
- When listening to music, try to identify the instruments that are being played.
- Make a list of the smells that you recall from your childhood.
- Sit outside and make a list of as many sounds as you can.
- Sit in a room and make a list of all of the things that you see, from a fly on the wall to the wall itself.
- Think of your favorite meal and imagine all of the tastes.
- Minimize your intake of alcohol.
- Cut down on your sugar intake.
- Try new recipes and foods. Eat at ethnic restaurants. Pay close attention to the foods and how they taste.
- Undertake new projects that require you to touch, such as gardening, cooking, and building things.
- When trying to learn the name of a new person you've met, study how he or she looks and sounds, how his or her hair might feel, or whether he or she is wearing a particular cologne or perfume.
- Eat a meal blindfolded and try to identify each food by taste and smell alone.
- Make a list of the sights, sounds, tastes, smells, and touches that are associated with each of the four seasons.
- Take an imaginary trip to a baseball game and describe what you might taste, see, hear, smell, and touch.
- Think of your favorite song. Which senses does the song evoke? Were you with a special person when you first heard it? Were you at a particular place? Were there particular smells in the area? Were you eating a meal at the time?
- Plant a garden full of vegetables and beautiful flowers with wonderful smells. Spend time there.
- Hang bird feeders in your yard to watch the birds eat and listen to them sing.
- Open windows and let in outside smells, such as freshly mowed grass.
- Use aromatherapy.

Strengthen Your Mind Program: A Course for Memory Enhancement by Einberger & Sellick.

123

Musical Instruments

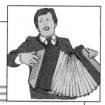

How many different types of musical instruments can you name? Think about how the instruments look, feel, and sound. Are there any that have a particular smell or are maybe associated with a certain smell? For example, an accordion might remind you of the taste and smell of German food, the feel of air going in and out, a person dressed in traditional German attire, or the sounds of polka music!

1.

2.

3.

4.

5.

6.

7.

8.

9.

10.

11.

12.

13.

14.

15.

Strengthen Your Mind Program: A Course for Memory Enhancement by Einberger & Sellick.
© 2010 by Health Professions Press, Inc.

Morning Time

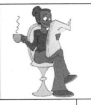

Think of the senses you use when you wake up each morning and prepare for your day. This is a time when all of the senses come alive! What are some things that awaken each of your senses first thing in the morning?

Sense of sight

Sense of hearing

Sense of touch

Sense of smell

Sense of taste

Grocery Store Scavenger Hunt

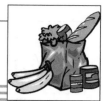

Grocery stores can be a great place to use all of your senses. Take a trip to your local store to identify the following items. If this is not possible, use magazines, newspapers, or simply your imagination to complete the exercise. Whichever way, you're sure to bring up many memories associated with food!

Two items that you could identify by touch alone (e.g., a clove of garlic).
    1.
    2.

Two items that have a sour taste.
    1.
    2.

Two items that you could identify by smell alone (e.g., a lemon).
    1.
    2.

Two items (not in the produce section) that are red.
    1.
    2.

Two items that are soft.
    1.
    2.

Two items that make a fairly loud noise when eaten.
    1.
    2.

Two fruits that have a strong smell.
    1.
    2.

Two vegetables with a strong smell.
    1.
    2.

Two items that are sticky.
    1.
    2.

Strengthen Your Mind Program: A Course for Memory Enhancement by Einberger & Sellick.
© 2010 by Health Professions Press, Inc.

Well-Known Advertisements

The advertisements below relate in some way to one or more of the five senses. Can you name the product?

1. Nothin' says lovin' like somethin' from the oven.

2. When it rains, it pours.

3. You're in good hands.

4. We'll leave the light on for you.

5. Fly the friendly skies.

6. M'mm, m'mm good.

7. Good to the last drop.

8. It keeps going and going . . .

9. Snap, crackle, pop.

10. Double your pleasure, double your fun.

11. Breakfast of champions.

12. America's most favorite dessert.

13. Let your fingers do the walking.

14. Please don't squeeze the _____.

15. The instrument of the immortals.

16. Melts in your mouth, not in your hands.

17. _____ fights bad breath.

18. The pause that refreshes.

Well-Known Advertisements ANSWER SHEET

1. Nothin' says lovin' like somethin' from the oven.   **Pillsbury**

2. When it rains, it pours.   **Morton Salt**

3. You're in good hands.   **Allstate**

4. We'll leave the light on for you.   **Motel 6**

5. Fly the friendly skies.   **United Airlines**

6. M'mm, m'mm good.   **Campbell's Soup**

7. Good to the last drop.   **Maxwell House**

8. It keeps going and going . . .   **Energizer Bunny (Energizer batteries)**

9. Snap, crackle, pop.   **Rice Krispies**

10. Double your pleasure, double your fun.   **Doublemint Gum**

11. Breakfast of champions.   **Wheaties**

12. America's most favorite dessert.   **Jell-O**

13. Let your fingers do the walking.   **Yellow Pages**

14. Please don't squeeze the _____.   **Charmin**

15. The instrument of the immortals.   **Steinway & Sons**

16. Melts in your mouth, not in your hands.   **M&M's**

17. _____ fights bad breath.   **Listerine**

18. The pause that refreshes.   **Coca-Cola**

Strengthen Your Mind Program: A Course for Memory Enhancement by Einberger & Sellick.

Stress

Stress
FACILITATOR OVERVIEW

For all of us stress is a part of daily life. Driving to work, dealing with an unpleasant encounter with another person, handling money or health issues—these situations all require some level of response. The feeling of stress is what encourages us to respond. Too much stress is bad in many ways; it affects the body, mind, and general health. Did you know, however, that too little stress is not good either?

This lesson focuses on the causes of stress, the difference between good and bad stress, tips for managing stress, and how stress affects memory. As we grow older and stress becomes more and more a part of our lives, it is important that we develop tools to manage stressful situations. Practicing stress management techniques can help to keep the body and mind healthy and not allow stress to affect memory.

HOW STRESS AFFECTS US

Numerous studies have documented the effects of stress on the body. Stress can raise your blood pressure, lower your immune system, raise your resting heart rate, and make you feel nervous or faint. In addition, you may feel tightness in your shoulders or neck area and have shallow breathing, headaches, stomachaches, or general pain. Some people feel overly tired when they are stressed, while others feel energetic or jittery.

Too much stress can also affect your mental and emotional health. You may have trouble focusing, feel depressed, have difficulty with everyday decisions, or feel helpless. Some people may view and treat themselves very negatively in response to stress and may have difficulty enjoying their usual interests.

Researchers have also found that short- and long-term stress can have negative impacts on the brain and memory. According to a study conducted by Latham (2007), stress that lasts as little as a few hours can impair brain-cell communication in areas associated with learning and memory. The study also found that acute stress activates select molecules that impair the memory collection and storage process in the brain. According to a study reported by the University of California at Irvine (2008), stress causes stress hormones in the brain to divert energy from the hippocampus (the area of the brain that is central to learning and memory) to areas that need it more. This decrease in available energy compromises the brain's ability to create new memories, which explains why a person who has experienced a traumatic event, such as a car accident or robbery, often feels confused or forgets details of the event or the event in its entirety.

Chronic or long-term stress can cause you to feel out of control of your life. Renowned researcher Robert M. Sapolsky found that long-term, chronic stress can damage the hippocampus. Too much stress causes the brain to release stress hormones that adversely affect memory. The main culprit in this case is the stress hormone cortisol, too much of which can prevent the brain from forming new memories or from recalling existing memories.

GOOD STRESS VERSUS BAD STRESS

Although too much stress is bad for us, the good news is that not all stress is bad. According to Janata (2009), both good stress (called *eustress*) and bad stress (*distress*) challenge us. Eustress is what makes us get up in the morning and get ready for a meeting or appointment. Eustress is also what you may feel before a job interview or sports activity—it gives you the energy that you need to be successful at what you need or want to do. Without eustress, or good stress, life would be boring and unexciting. More important, without good stress you may not live up to your potential or challenge yourself.

When stress becomes overwhelming (and the rate at which it becomes unmanageable is different for everybody), it becomes distress, which interferes with daily life and can cause you to feel out of control and helpless. On their Web site, the Mountain State Centers for Independent Living lists the following facts about distress:

- Millions of Americans suffer from stress each year.

- Three out of four people say they experience stress at least twice a month.

- More than half of those people say they suffer from "high" levels of stress at least twice a month.

- From 1988 to 2008, the number of people who reported that stress affects their work quadrupled.

- One-fourth of all drugs prescribed in the United States are for the treatment of stress.

MANAGING STRESS IN DAILY LIFE

One of the most important things that you can do for your emotional, physical, and cognitive health is to control or try to reduce the amount of stress you experience on a daily basis.

Below are 10 tips to feel more in control and less stressed. (Discuss these tips with participants as well as those that are a part of the handouts *Stress Reducers* and *Dealing with Stress—The Fours As*.)

1. Use a calendar to schedule important things. Give items a date and a priority.

2. Create lists to keep track of things that need to be done. Even if it is a long list, crossing items off can help you feel accomplished.

3. Practice yoga, guided imagery, or meditation to relax and calm your mind.

4. Ask yourself how important something truly is to you. Maybe you are feeling stress over something that you are better off letting go.

5. Delegate to family, friends, or coworkers, and don't be afraid to ask for help.

6. Exercise regularly to burn off extra stress hormones.

7. Get enough sleep so that you feel recharged and refreshed.

8. Eat well and reduce your caffeine and sugar intake.

9. Stay socially active. Share your successes, concerns, and issues with friends and family.

10. Give yourself at least 10 minutes to relax every day.

Stress
FACILITATOR INSTRUCTIONS

1.   WELCOME AND INTRODUCTION (15 MINUTES)

To do before class:

- Read and familiarize yourself with the Stress Overview.
- Write the following quote on a board or flip chart.

> "Without the resistance of the wind, an eagle would never fly."
> (Unknown)

- Familiarize yourself with and make appropriate copies of the warm-up activity, quiz, practice activities, and homework.

Greet the participants and make introductions, if necessary. Tell them that the topic of the class is stress and how it can affect memory. Ask participants to think of a recent time when they felt stressed. (Ask them to think about their stressful situation for a discussion later on in the class.) Explain that stress has a negative effect on the body and that too much stress is bad for memory as well.

Discuss the quote and ask participants for their interpretations. Ask them how they perceive the stress in their lives (how does stress affect them physically or mentally?).

2.   WARM-UP ACTIVITY (10 MINUTES)

Ask participants to break into groups of two or three. Then ask them to take turns sharing their recent stressful situation with the group and to explain how the situation affected them physically and mentally (if they are not comfortable with this, they do not have to share). Finally, ask participants to share how the situation was resolved or, if it is not yet resolved, to brainstorm ideas with the group.

Give the groups 5 minutes to discuss and brainstorm ideas. Then bring the entire class back together and spend 5 minutes having volunteers share their stressful situations with the whole group. After several people have spoken, explain that by sharing their experiences with others, everyone in the room will hopefully have decreased their level of stress and increased their ability to cope with their stressful situation.

3.   STRESS QUIZ (10 MINUTES)

Pass out the *Stress Quiz* and explain to participants that this exercise is something for fun, that it doesn't matter how well or poorly they do. If they are unsure of an answer, they should feel free to not respond (or to give their best guess!). Give participants about 5 minutes to complete the quiz and then go over the answers as a group.

4. EXPLANATION AND DISCUSSION OF STRESS AND HOW IT AFFECTS MEMORY (15 MINUTES)

Explain how stress affects us (physically and mentally), talk about good stress versus bad stress, and review the stress management techniques. Pause periodically to ask if anyone has questions or comments.

5. PRACTICE ACTIVITIES (30 MINUTES)

Pass out the *Stress Self-Assessment*, and allow participants about 5 minutes to complete it. Explain that the assessment will give participants the opportunity to reflect on the stress in their lives. After they have finished, ask participants how they scored. Did anyone have an especially low or high score? Did anyone find something in the assessment that they hadn't realized was making them feel stressed? Ask for someone with a low score to share his or her stress management tips.

Distribute the handout *Stress Reducers*. Explain that one of the best ways to maintain good health is to learn and practice stress management. Review each stress reducer and ask for feedback as well as for personal experiences from those who have tried any of the techniques. Ask participants to share techniques that are not included in the list that they use to manage stress.

Pass out the worksheet *Managing Stress*. Ask participants to list one or two primary sources of stress in their lives. Then ask them to list what, if anything, they could change about the source of their stress as well as steps that they could take to manage the stressor. After about 5 minutes, ask participants to share some of the tips that they listed for reducing or managing stress.

6. REVIEW AND CLOSING (5 MINUTES)

Thank the group for their participation and ask them to try at least one new stress management technique this week. Encourage them to take steps to reduce their overall stress and to be aware of the effect that stress can have on memory. Finally, end the class with a deep-breathing exercise. Ask the group to sit up in their chairs with both feet on the floor. Tell them to close their eyes and take one deep breath in. Ask them to blow the breath out through their nose and repeat five times. Remind them that they can do this exercise anywhere and at any time of the day.

7. HOMEWORK (5 MINUTES)

Pass out the homework sheets and explain what should be done for each. Remind participants that homework should be fun, and encourage them to enlist the help of family and friends or to use resources such as the Internet.

- *Famous Scandals* (Ask the group to think about the stress level of the people involved in these scandals!)
- *Stress Reducers A–Z*
- *Dealing with Stress—The Four As*
- *Healthy Ways to Relax and Recharge*
- Practice managing stress in your life and really try to reduce at least one area of stress!

Stress
CLASS AGENDA

1. Welcome and Introduction
2. Warm-Up Activity
   - A Stressful Situation (Group Activity)
3. *Stress Quiz*
4. Overview of Stress and How It Affects the Mind, Body, and Memory
   - How Stress Affects Us
   - Good Stress versus Bad Stress
   - Managing Stress in Daily Life
5. Practice Activities
   - *Stress Self-Assessment*
   - *Stress Reducers*
   - *Managing Stress*
6. Review and Closing
7. Homework (fun, not stressful!)
   - *Famous Scandals*
   - *Stress Reducers A–Z*
   - *Dealing with Stress—The Four As*
   - *Healthy Ways to Relax and Recharge*
   - Practice managing stress in your life, and really try to reduce at least one area of stress!

Strengthen Your Mind Program: A Course for Memory Enhancement by Einberger & Sellick.

Stress Quiz

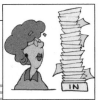

1. Some immediate symptoms of stress are
   A. Sweating
   B. Rapid heartbeat
   C. Change in appetite
   D. Acne
   E. All of the above

2. Some long-term symptoms of stress are
   A. Fatigue
   B. Inability to concentrate
   C. Irritability
   D. Depression
   E. Headaches
   F. All of the above

3. Stress can be dangerous when
   A. It makes you irritable toward friends
   B. It gives you butterflies in your stomach
   C. It makes you crave chocolate
   D. It interferes with your ability to live a normal life

4. Stress can age a person by
   A. Creating wrinkles and gray hair
   B. Raising blood pressure
   C. Affecting the immune system in ways that lead to heart disease, arthritis, diabetes, and other diseases
   D. All of the above

5. Stress is the body's way of
   A. Reacting to what seems like a threat
   B. Getting even for too much hard living
   C. Making sure that you don't overload yourself
   D. All of the above

6. True or False: *Short-term stress* refers to feeling stressed for a week or more.

7. True or False: Long-term stress is good for your brain because it forces your brain to focus more than it would otherwise.

8. What percentage of prescribed drugs in the United States goes toward the treatment of stress?
   A. 10%
   B. 25%
   C. 50%
   D. 75%

9. Which of the following is not a good way to manage stress?
   A. Have a strong social network of friends and family
   B. Exercise regularly
   C. Drink several alcoholic beverages each day
   D. Use tools to keep organized (such as a calendar)

10. True or False: Stress generally increases as a person gets older.

Stress Quiz ANSWER SHEET

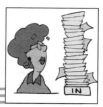

1. **Some immediate symptoms of stress are**
   E.   All of the above

2. **Some long-term symptoms of stress are**
   F.   All of the above

3. **Stress can be dangerous when**
   D.   It interferes with your ability to live a normal life

4. **Stress can age a person by**
   D.   All of the above

5. **Stress is the body's way of**
   A.   Reacting to what seems like a threat

6. **True or False: *Short-term stress* refers to feeling stressed for a week or more.**
   False

7. **True or False: Long-term stress is good for your brain because it forces your brain to focus more than it would otherwise.**
   False

8. **What percentage of prescribed drugs in the United States goes toward the treatment of stress?**
   B.   25%

9. **Which of the following is not a good way to manage stress?**
   C.   Drink several alcoholic beverages each day

10. **True or False: Stress generally increases as a person gets older.**
    True

Stress Self-Assessment

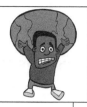

Check all of the stressors that apply to you.

— A recent illness

— A divorce or separation

— Family problems

— Spouse or partner ill or stressed

— Recent death of a loved one

— Loneliness

— Moving to a new location

— Weight gain or loss

— Being in debt

— Feeling overwhelmed

— Relationship problems

— Worrying about our society

— Unemployed

— New job

— Job stress/problems

— Anniversary of loved one's death

— Money issues

— Being hospitalized

— Legal problems

— Friend/family with substance abuse

— Transportation problems

— Going back to work

— Holidays

— Neighbors are too loud

— Medication issues

— Sleeping problems

— Lack of education

— Feeling isolated

— Worrying about appearances

— Wanting to eat but on a diet

— Someone telling you what to do

— Threat of war

— Violence in neighborhood

— Lack of recreation involvement

— Boredom

— Depression

— Anxiety

— Mental health issues

— Unresolved family issues

— Change in living situation

— Making new friends

— Needing to borrow money

— Anger issues

— Not enough time

— Too much time

— Waiting in a long line

— Dealing with the medical establishment

— Substance abuse problems

— Starting a new relationship

— Change in family member's health

— Going back to school

— Change in financial status

— Falling in love

— Sexual problems

— Motivation problems

— Unable to relax

— Worrying a lot

NUMBER OF CHECKS _____

0–20   Mild stress

21–40   Moderate stress

41+   Extreme stress

Strengthen Your Mind Program: A Course for Memory Enhancement by Einberger & Sellick.
© 2010 by Health Professions Press, Inc.

Stress Reducers

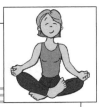

- Allow 15 minutes of extra time to get to appointments.
- Eliminate or reduce the amount of caffeine in your diet.
- Always set up contingency plans just in case. ("If we get separated at the shopping center, here's where we'll meet.")
- Organize your life.
- Simplify, simplify, simplify.
- Make friends with "nonworriers." Nothing can get you into the habit of worrying faster than associating with chronic worrywarts.
- Get enough sleep. If necessary, use an alarm clock to remind you to go to bed!
- Writing down your thoughts and feelings in a journal or on paper can help you to clarify things.
- Talk it out. Discussing your problems with a trusted friend or relative can help to clear your mind of confusion so that you can concentrate on problem solving.
- Learn to live one day at a time.
- Every day do something you really enjoy. Nurture yourself.
- Add an ounce of love to everything you do.
- Take a hot bath or shower to relieve tension.
- Eliminate destructive "self-talk." ("I'm too old to . . . ," "I'm too fat to . . . ," etc.)
- Do one thing at a time.
- Every day allow yourself time for privacy, quiet, and introspection.
- Have an optimistic view of the world. Believe that most people are doing the best they can.
- When you feel that stress is building up within you, if possible, stop what you are doing and take a short walk.
- Practice deep breathing.
- Listen to your favorite music.
- Increase your social outlets.
- Spend time in a garden or gardening.
- Watch a funny movie. Use humor every day.
- Engage in some sort of sport or physical activity.
- Read a good book.
- Make your favorite meal or eat your favorite food.
- Practice meditation and/or guided imagery.
- Eat a well-balanced diet.

Managing Stress

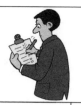

List one or two primary sources of stress for you.

1.

2.

Can you change anything about these stressors? If so, what?

What actions can you take to reduce or manage stress?

1.

2.

3.

4.

5.

Famous Scandals

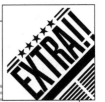

Scandals seem to be a staple of the political and entertainment world. Listed below are the descriptions of many well-known incidents where people had the "wool pulled over their eyes." Match the description on the left with the name on the right.

___ 1. In the 1950s, it was revealed that several popular television quiz shows were secretly rigged by producers.

___ 2. Orson Wells directed an adaptation of this novel that aired on October 30, 1968, causing many to believe that an actual alien invasion was taking place in the United States.

___ 3. This well-known political scandal took place in 1972 in Washington, DC, and led to the resignation of President Nixon.

___ 4. In this famous archaeological hoax, pieces of bone believed to be that of an early human were, over 40 years later, discovered to be that of a modern man and an orangutan.

___ 5. This Texas-based energy company was once considered one of the most innovative, successful companies to work for, until it was forced into bankruptcy by a major accounting fraud.

___ 6. This famous televangelist and minister was convicted of accounting fraud for misusing hundreds of thousands of dollars in donations given to his popular ministry in the 1980s.

___ 7. During the Reagan Administration, this political scandal involved selling weapons to Iran and using the profits to fund anti-communist rebels.

___ 8. In the 1990s, this famous filmmaker came under scrutiny for having a relationship with his long-time girlfriend's adopted daughter, whom he later married.

___ 9. This famous scandal took place under President Harding in 1921 and involved a navy oil reserve being secretly leased to a private company.

___ 10. The 1919 World Series resulted in this famous baseball scandal involving eight players who attempted to "fix" the game.

___ 11. In this Hollywood scandal, actors Debbie Reynolds and Eddie Fisher ended their marriage when it was revealed that Fisher fell in love with whom?

___ 12. In 1875, it was revealed that a group of distillers and public officials were stealing the proceeds of over-inflated taxes on liquor.

___ 13. Some say that there are still sightings of this famous rock star who died in 1977, leading many to say that he faked his own death.

a. Enron

b. Elvis Presley

c. Black Sox Scandal

d. Quiz Show Scandals

e. Iran Contra Affair

f. Watergate

g. The Whiskey Ring

h. Elizabeth Taylor

i. *War of the Worlds*

j. Piltdown Man

k. Jim Bakker

l. Woody Allen

m. Teapot Dome

Famous Scandals ANSWER SHEET

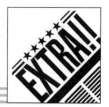

1. In the 1950s, it was revealed that several popular television quiz shows were secretly rigged by producers.

   d. Quiz Show Scandals

2. Orson Wells directed an adaptation of this novel that aired on October 30, 1968, causing many to believe that an actual alien invasion was taking place in the United States.

   i. *War of the Worlds*

3. This well-known political scandal took place in 1972 in Washington, DC, and led to the resignation of President Nixon.

   f. Watergate

4. In this famous archaeological hoax, pieces of bone believed to be that of an early human were, over 40 years later, discovered to be that of a modern man and an orangutan.

   j. Piltdown man

5. This Texas-based energy company was once considered one of the most innovative, successful companies to work for, until it was forced into bankruptcy by a major accounting fraud.

   a. Enron

6. This famous televangelist and minister was convicted of accounting fraud for misusing hundreds of thousands of dollars in donations given to his popular ministry in the 1980s.

   k. Jim Bakker

7. During the Reagan Administration, this political scandal involved selling weapons to Iran and using the profits to fund anti-communist rebels.

   e. Iran Contra Affair

8. In the 1990s, this famous filmmaker came under scrutiny for having a relationship with his long-time girlfriend's adopted daughter, whom he later married.

   l. Woody Allen

9. This famous scandal took place under President Harding in 1921 and involved a navy oil reserve being secretly leased to a private company.

   m. Teapot Dome

10. The 1919 World Series resulted in this famous baseball scandal involving eight players who attempted to "fix" the game.

    c. Black Sox Scandal

11. In this Hollywood scandal, actors Debbie Reynolds and Eddie Fisher ended their marriage when it was revealed that Fisher fell in love with whom?

    h. Elizabeth Taylor

12. In 1875, it was revealed that a group of distillers and public officials were stealing the proceeds of over-inflated taxes on liquor.

    g. The Whiskey Ring

13. Some say that there are still sightings of this famous rock star who died in 1977, leading many to say that he faked his own death.

    b. Elvis Presley

Reprinted from *Strengthen Your Mind, Volume Two* by Einberger & Sellick.

Stress Reducers A–Z

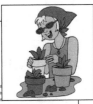

Think of a creative way to reduce stress that begins with each letter of the alphabet.

A

B

C

D

E

F

G

H

I

J

K

L

M

N

O

P

Q

R

S

T

U

V

W

X

Y

Z

Strengthen Your Mind Program: A Course for Memory Enhancement by Einberger & Sellick.

Dealing with Stress—The Four As

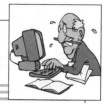

Change the stressor—*Avoid* the situation or *Alter* the situation.

Change your reaction—*Adapt* to the stressor or *Accept* the stressor.

1. *Avoid* the situation.
   - Learn to say no.
   - Avoid people who stress you out.
   - Take control of your environment.
   - Avoid hot-button topics.
   - Pare down your to-do list.

2. *Alter* the situation.
   - Express your feelings instead of keeping them to yourself.
   - Be willing to compromise.
   - Be more assertive.
   - Manage your time.

3. *Adapt* to the stressor.
   - Reframe your problems.
   - Look at the big picture.
   - Adjust your standards.
   - Focus on the positive.

4. *Accept* the stressor.
   - Don't try to control the uncontrollable.
   - Look for the upside.
   - Share your feelings.
   - Learn to forgive.

Additional ways to deal with stress.
   - Set aside relaxation time.
   - Connect with others.
   - Do something you enjoy every day.
   - Keep your sense of humor.

Strengthen Your Mind Program: A Course for Memory Enhancement by Einberger & Sellick.

Healthy Ways to Relax and Recharge

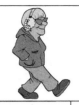

Below are several healthy ways that you can relax and recharge your mind, body, and memory. On the lines at the bottom, list five other ways that you can relax and recharge.

Go for a walk.

Spend time in nature.

Call a good friend.

Sweat out tension with a good workout.

Write in a journal.

Take a long bath.

Light scented candles.

Savor a warm cup of coffee or tea.

Play with a pet.

Work in your garden.

Get a massage.

Listen to music.

Watch a comedy show.

_____

_____

_____

_____

_____

Optimism and Humor

Optimism and Humor
FACILITATOR OVERVIEW

The *American Heritage College Dictionary* defines *optimism* as "a tendency to expect the best possible outcome or dwell on the most hopeful aspects of a situation." An *optimist* is "one who usually expects a favorable outcome." *Humor* is defined as "that which is intended to induce laughter or amusement." Optimism and humor are qualities that can and do have a significant impact on one's memory.

BENEFITS OF OPTIMISM

There are many benefits of optimism, including the following:

- Reduced stress

- Decreased likelihood of depression

- Better health

- Increased self-esteem

- Greater likelihood of achieving goals and dreams

- Quicker recovery from setbacks

- Longer life expectancy

- Increased sense of life satisfaction.

- Greater likelihood of having healthy relationships.

Research has shown that optimistic people also have better memories. If you believe that you'll be able to remember something, you'll be more likely to remember than if you had the pessimistic attitude of "I'm never going to remember that." Recall the children's book *The Little Engine That Could* (Piper, 1976). The book is used to teach children about the value of optimism and hard work. In the tale, a long train must be pulled over a mountain. Various larger engines are asked to pull the train, but for different reasons they refuse. Finally, a small engine agrees to try and succeeds in pulling the train over the mountain, all the while repeating over and over "I think I can, I think I can, I think I can." It believed that it could, and indeed did, pull the longer train over the mountain by maintaining a positive, optimistic attitude.

MAKING LEMONADE OUT OF LIFE'S LEMONS

In his book *Aging Well: Surprising Guideposts to a Happier Life*, Dr. George E. Vaillant analyzes data from three separate longevity studies involving more than 800 individuals—

men and women, rich and poor—who were followed for more than 50 years, from adolescence to old age (2002). Dr. Vaillant found that one of the most powerful predictors of successful aging is habitually using coping mechanisms or defenses that "make lemonade out of life's lemons." Dr. Vaillant's study identified the following five coping mechanisms (Martinuzzi, 2006):

- Altruism (doing for others what they need, not what we want to do for them)

- Sublimation (diverting energy to more constructive pursuits, such as creativity, art, sports)

- Suppression (postponement, not repression, of stressors)

- Humor

- Anticipation (realistic, hopeful planning for the future; not operating in a pessimistic crisis mode, but preparing and adapting for whatever life brings).

Optimism isn't necessarily an inborn trait; it can be learned and nurtured. The handout *How Can We Nurture Optimism?* lists ways that we can do just that.

BENEFITS OF HUMOR AND LAUGHTER

Just as optimism has an effect on memory, so do humor and laughter. The benefits of humor and laughter include:

- Are relaxing and help to relieve stress

- Nurture optimism

- Reduce anxiety, fear, and anger

- Exercise the chest muscles and lungs

- Help to control pain by distraction (focusing "outside the body") and through an increased production of endorphins (the body's natural painkiller)

- Lower blood pressure

- Improve mood

- Promote an overall sense of well-being and increased self-esteem.

As with optimism, the benefits of humor and laughter can result in improved memory when they are a regular, frequent part of an individual's life. Unfortunately, as we get older, we laugh much less frequently than children. On average 5-year-olds laugh between 400–450 times a day, whereas adults laugh only 12–20 times a day. With increased responsibilities and greater individual and societal pressures, it would be expected that adults would laugh less than children—but so much less? The reason for the drastic difference is a good topic for discussion.

We can all learn to add more humor and laughter into our everyday lives. The handout *Incorporate Humor into Everyday Life* is a good starting point for discussing ways to do so.

Optimism and Humor
FACILITATOR INSTRUCTIONS

1. WELCOME AND INTRODUCTION (10 MINUTES)

To do before class:

- Read and familiarize yourself with the Optimism and Humor Overview.

- Write the following quotes on a board or flip chart:

> "A pessimist sees the difficulty in every opportunity; an optimist
> sees the opportunity in every difficulty."
> (Winston Churchill, British Prime Minister)

> "The average pencil is seven inches long with just a half-inch eraser—
> in case you thought optimism was dead."
> (Robert Brault, freelance writer)

- Familiarize yourself with and make appropriate copies of the warm-up activity, quiz, handouts, practice activities, and homework.

Welcome participants and make introductions, if necessary. Explain that the class will focus on optimism and humor and their relationship to memory. Read to participants the definitions of *optimism*, *optimist*, and *humor* given in the overview. Ask participants if they believe that optimism and humor can have a profound impact on memory and how. Discuss the quotes and ask participants for their interpretations.

2. WARM-UP ACTIVITY (10 MINUTES)

Pass out the worksheet *Happiness*. Give the group 4–5 minutes to complete it. When everyone is done, ask participants to share some of the things that make them happy. Encourage them to consider the things that make others in the class happy and perhaps add some of them to their own list.

3. QUIZ (10 MINUTES)

Pass out the quiz *How Optimistic Are You?* Give everyone 5 minutes to complete it. Although there's no special scoring for this quiz, it's a good way for participants to consider their level of optimism and how it affects their lives. Ask them if there are areas that they would like to improve. How many consider themselves to be optimists? Pessimists?

4. EXPLANATION AND DISCUSSION OF OPTIMISM AND HUMOR AND HOW THEY AFFECT MEMORY (30 MINUTES)

Explain how what we think affects how we feel. Discuss the benefits of optimism and the differences between an optimist and a pessimist. Review the benefits of humor and laughter. Distribute the handout *How Can We Nurture Optimism?* Review the list, asking for feedback from the class as you go along. Ask them for tips to add to the list. Next, distribute the handout *Incorporate Humor into Everyday Life*. Review the suggestions as a group, again asking for additions to the list.

5. PRACTICE ACTIVITIES (20 MINUTES)

After learning new ways to nurture optimism and to incorporate humor into everyday life, the group will next have the opportunity to practice nurturing optimism.

Pass out the worksheet *Ways to Show Appreciation and Thanks* and have participants work on it individually or in small groups. After completion, brainstorm with the entire group the many ways to show appreciation and thanks.

Next, divide participants into two groups. Pass out the worksheet *Turn a Pessimistic Statement into a Positive One*. Give the groups 5 minutes to complete the task and then review as a whole group. Let participants know that the technique can be used often and encourage them to practice. Possible answers for the practice activity could be:

- I don't have to water the grass.
- I can use my new umbrella.
- There may be a beautiful rainbow after the rain stops.
- I can stay inside and curl up with a good book.
- There won't be as many people at the grocery store when I go shopping later.
- The rain will wash off some of the dirt from my car.
- I'll be able to listen to the wonderful sound of rain on my roof.

6. REVIEW AND CLOSING (5 MINUTES)

Thank the group for their participation. Remind them how important an optimistic attitude is to having a good memory and that an optimistic attitude can be nurtured and strengthened. Ask participants to review the three handouts and to think of more additions to the lists. Ask them to review the quiz and think about how to answer *always* to most of the questions, rather than *sometimes* or *never*. Discuss the value of instilling more humor and laughter into their everyday lives and review ways to do so.

7. HOMEWORK (5 MINUTES)

Pass out the homework sheets and explain what should be done for each. Remind the group that it's important to practice what's been learned in class in order to better remember the information.

- *Nurturing Optimism*
- *Comedy, Laughter, and Smiles* (Three great ways to enhance optimism!)
- Remind participants to practice optimism, use more humor in everyday life, and laugh more often!

Optimism and Humor
CLASS AGENDA

1. Welcome and Introduction
2. Warm-Up Activity
   - *Happiness*
3. Quiz
   - *How Optimistic Are You?*
4. Optimism and Humor and Their Effect on Memory
   - *How Can We Nurture Optimism?*
   - *Incorporate Humor into Everyday Life*
5. Practice Activities
   - *Ways to Show Appreciation and Thanks*
   - *Turn a Pessimistic Statement into a Positive One*
6. Review and Closing
7. Homework
   - *Nurturing Optimism*
   - *Comedy, Laughter, and Smiles*
   - Practice optimism, use more humor in your everyday life, and laugh more often!

Strengthen Your Mind Program: A Course for Memory Enhancement by Einberger & Sellick.

Happiness

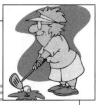

Reflect on those things that make you happy, bring a smile to your face, or make you laugh. List ten of those things below.

1.

2.

3.

4.

5.

6.

7.

8.

9.

10.

How Optimistic Are You?

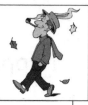

Never Sometimes Always

1. I look for the positive in situations.

2. I see the best in people rather than focusing on their faults.

3. I focus on my strengths rather than my weaknesses.

4. I see my weak areas as challenges to work on rather than faults that cannot be overcome.

5. I do not use alcohol or drugs to deal with difficult times.

6. I limit the time I spend with pessimistic people.

7. I try to surround myself with optimistic people.

8. I see mistakes as opportunities to learn and grow.

9. I believe that I *can* improve my memory.

10. I often use humor to get me through difficult times.

11. I believe that, in general, life is good.

12. I believe that my level of optimism has a direct impact on my physical health.

13. I spend time with people who make me laugh.

14. I believe that negativity can adversely affect my memory.

15. I know that if I *believe* that I can do or remember something, I am more likely to succeed in doing so.

16. When I have a problem, I try to solve it rather than merely complain about it.

17. I am flexible.

18. I try to focus on what I can control rather than what I have no control over.

Strengthen Your Mind Program: A Course for Memory Enhancement by Einberger & Sellick.

How Can We Nurture Optimism?

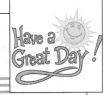

Attitude is your choice—think positive! Here are some tips for a positive attitude. Feel free to compile your own list of additional tips.

- Look for the best in every situation.

- Focus on what you can control rather than what is out of your control.

- Know your strengths and celebrate them! Focus on what you do well.

- Learn from your mistakes. Plan a different way to handle a situation the next time.

- Spend time solving a problem rather than focusing on complaining about it.

- Find the positive in all that surrounds you.

- Incorporate more humor and laughter into your daily life.

- Look at tough times as learning experiences.

- Seek out the positive and make a conscious effort to enjoy life.

- Develop relationships and connect with others who are optimistic.

- Decrease the time you spend with pessimistic people and/or in negative environments.

- Volunteer. The chance to do something meaningful for others creates joy.

- Change your language. Get rid of the "buts"—they can negate what you said before the "but." For example, change "I love the rain, *but* it means I can't take a walk today" to "I love the rain, *and* I think I'll need to exercise inside today."

- Focus "outside" of yourself on family, friends, projects, possibilities— things that are exciting to you.

- Celebrate each day!

Strengthen Your Mind Program: A Course for Memory Enhancement by Einberger & Sellick.
© 2010 by Health Professions Press, Inc.

Incorporate Humor into Everyday Life

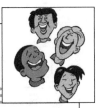

Humor and laughter have a multitude of benefits, including lowering blood pressure, improving mood and spirit, relieving stress, nurturing optimism, and improving one's memory! There are many ways to incorporate humor into everyday life. Try some of the following and watch your outlook improve!

- Schedule fun into your day. Plan to do at least one fun thing every day. Don't wait for fun to happen on its own.

- Smile at yourself or someone else for no reason!

- Watch or play with children or with pets.

- Learn and tell jokes.

- Watch funny movies.

- Read cartoons.

- Listen to old radio shows.

- Keep a humor file of funny cartoons, stories, pictures, buttons, bumper stickers, and so forth.

- Surround yourself with humorous people.

- Read a humorous novel or book of short stories.

- Give your enthusiasm to everyone. See the funny side of life.

- Alter your attitude!

 Strengthen Your Mind Program: A Course for Memory Enhancement by Einberger & Sellick.
© 2010 by Health Professions Press, Inc.

Ways to Show Appreciation and Thanks

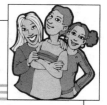

Name as many ways that you can think of to show appreciation and thanks. They can include phrases in foreign languages!

1.

2.

3.

4.

5.

6.

7.

8.

9.

10.

11.

12.

13.

14.

15.

16.

17.

18.

Strengthen Your Mind Program: A Course for Memory Enhancement by Einberger & Sellick.
© 2010 by Health Professions Press, Inc.

Turn a Pessimistic Statement into a Positive One

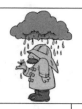

Turn the following pessimistic statement into an optimistic one by listing five things that are positive about the situation.

"I am so upset because it's raining today. Now I can't go for the long walk I wanted to take."

1.

2.

3.

4.

5.

Strengthen Your Mind Program: A Course for Memory Enhancement by Einberger & Sellick.

Nurturing Optimism

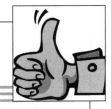

Pick three things from the *How Can We Nurture Optimism?* list and practice them in the coming months. Then choose three more and so on. Study the list and add your own ideas. Be willing to try those that you don't think will work. You may be surprised!

1.

2.

3.

Comedy, Laughter, and Smiles

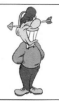

Laughter is a universal language. It does wonderful things for our bodies and our minds. The following activity deals with laughter and comedy in a variety of ways. How many people, phrases, or words can you identify?

1. These comic performers usually wear colored wigs, outlandish costumes, face paint, and a round red nose.

2. Often heard on television, this soundtrack is made up of the sounds of audience laughter.

3. A laugh that involves much of the body, especially the stomach, is called a what?

4. This comedian traveled the globe during the holidays to entertain U.S. troops for nearly 6 decades.

5. A humorous drawing often with a caption included is called a what?

6. Freddy the Freeloader and Clem Kadiddlehopper were two of this comedian's most famous characters.

7. This comedian was famous for her reporting of American home life in the last half of the 20th century. Her second-favorite household chore was ironing. Her first was hitting her head on the top bunk bed until she fainted.

8. This type of comedy often involves some kind of physical activity, such as that used frequently by The Three Stooges.

9. "My wife Mary and I have been married for 47 years, and not once have we had an argument serious enough to consider divorce. Murder, yes, but divorce, never." This famous quote was made by this comedian about his wife, Mary Livingston.

10. This famous sex symbol was famous for her off-color quotes. She once said, "I generally avoid temptation unless I can't resist it."

11. This cigar-smoking, hard-living star hated "children, dogs, and women, unless they were the wrong sort of women."

12. This is the day of the year when many people trick one another with practical jokes.

13. This is the common name of the elbow and is also an expression defined as one's sense of humor.

14. "One of these days . . . POW, right in the kisser!" was one of this comedian's most famous lines (spoken to his TV wife, Alice).

15. "Heeeeeere's Johnny!" was the line spoken by Ed McMahon to introduce this man on *The Tonight Show*.

16. "God don't make no mistakes. That's how He got to be God." This is just one of the many famous quotes by this man, who was the star of *All in the Family* in the 1970s.

Reprinted from *Strengthen Your Mind, Volume Two* by Einberger & Sellick.

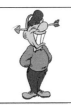

1. These comic performers usually wear colored wigs, outlandish costumes, face paint, and a round red nose.
   clowns

2. Often heard on television, this soundtrack is made up of the sounds of audience laughter.
   canned laughter (laugh track)

3. A laugh that involves much of the body, especially the stomach, is called a what?
   belly laugh

4. This comedian traveled the globe during the holidays to entertain U.S. troops for nearly 6 decades.
   Bob Hope

5. A humorous drawing often with a caption included is called a what?
   cartoon

6. Freddy the Freeloader and Clem Kadiddlehopper were two of this comedian's most famous characters.
   Red Skelton

7. This comedian was famous for her reporting of American home life in the last half of the 20th century. Her second-favorite household chore was ironing. Her first was hitting her head on the top bunk bed until she fainted.
   Erma Bombeck

8. This type of comedy often involves some kind of physical activity, such as that used frequently by The Three Stooges.
   slapstick

9. "My wife Mary and I have been married for 47 years, and not once have we had an argument serious enough to consider divorce. Murder, yes, but divorce, never." This famous quote was made by this comedian about his wife, Mary Livingston.
   Jack Benny

10. This famous sex symbol was famous for her off-color quotes. She once said, "I generally avoid temptation unless I can't resist it."
    Mae West

11. This cigar-smoking, hard-living star hated "children, dogs, and women, unless they were the wrong sort of women."
    W. C. Fields

12. This is the day of the year when many people trick one another with practical jokes.
    April 1 (April Fools' Day)

13. This is the common name of the elbow and is also an expression defined as one's sense of humor.
    funny bone

14. "One of these days . . . POW, right in the kisser!" was one of this comedian's most famous lines (spoken to his TV wife, Alice).
    Jackie Gleason

15. "Heeeeeere's Johnny!" was the line spoken by Ed McMahon to introduce this man on *The Tonight Show*.
    Johnny Carson

16. "God don't make no mistakes. That's how He got to be God." This is just one of the many famous quotes by this man, who was the star of *All in the Family* in the 1970s.
    Carroll O'Connor

Nutrition

Nutrition
FACILITATOR OVERVIEW

The topic of nutrition seems to show up everywhere: on the news, in magazines, as a discussion at the dinner table, even from well-meaning friends who enjoy giving "tips" on what you should or shouldn't eat. Almost every day research tells us something new about what is considered good, or not good, for us to eat. While we know that eating right is necessary for our bodies, what does research tell us about nutrition and its effect on memory? In this class participants will learn which foods can help to enhance memory and perhaps even stave off memory loss. In addition, they will learn how to incorporate more memory-friendly foods into their daily diets and how to make brain-healthy food choices.

ANTIOXIDANTS

One brain-healthy component of diet and nutrition is antioxidants, which are food compounds that are most commonly found in vitamins C and E and beta carotene, a form of vitamin A and what gives carrots their orange color. These chemicals rid the body of free radicals, which develop when the body metabolizes food as well as through daily exposure to the environment. Free radicals can damage cells. Antioxidants also reduce the oxidative damage to cells. Oxidation, which can be thought of as the biological equivalent to rusting, seems to contribute to aging and cognitive decline. According to Bauer (2008), antioxidants also help to improve blood flow to the brain. How can you tell if a food is high in antioxidants? Look at its color. Foods that are darker in pigment have higher levels of antioxidants. Fruits that are known to be high in antioxidants are prunes, raisins, blueberries, blackberries, strawberries, raspberries, plums, oranges, red grapes, and cherries. Vegetables that are high in antioxidants are kale, spinach, Brussels sprouts, alfalfa sprouts, broccoli, beets, red bell pepper, onions, corn, and eggplant.

Among the variety of foods that are rich in antioxidants, berries stand out as the superstars. According to Bauer (2008), all berries are high-healthy compounds called anthocyanins and flavanoids, which may help protect against the breakdown of brain cells. So, fill your plate and snack on strawberries, blueberries, blackberries, raspberries, and other berries!

OMEGA-3 FATTY ACIDS

Research on omega-3 fatty acids has found that they are an area of food nutrition that is vital for brain health. These fatty acids are most commonly found in certain types of fish, especially wild salmon, sardines, trout, whitefish, tuna, swordfish, and mackerel. One study assessed the eating habits over 9 years of 700 men and women with an average age of 76. The researchers found that participants who ate an average of 2.9 servings of fish each week had a 47% lower risk of developing dementia than those who ate between 1 and 2 servings of fish each week (Kage, 2006). This slower rate of decline gave study participants the memory and thinking ability of a person 3 years younger! Another study by Bauer (2008) found that people with the highest levels of omega-3 fats were significantly less likely to be diagnosed with dementia.

What if fish is not your favorite food choice? Try to eat at least one serving per week and also incorporate regularly into your diet flaxseeds, almonds, and walnuts, which are also high in omega-3 fatty acids.

DARK GREEN, LEAFY VEGETABLES

Mom was right when she said "Eat your vegetables!" Dark green, leafy vegetables such as spinach, kale, collard greens, mustard greens, and turnip greens are high in folic acid or folate. In addition, according to Jaffe-Gill et al. (2007), they are also high in B vitamins (B_6 and B_{12}), which are critical to keeping memory sharp. Australian research found that eating foods rich in folic acid is associated with faster processing of information and memory recall (Bauer, 2008).

One of the important benefits of folate is that it lowers the level of homocysteine in the blood. High levels of homocysteine have been associated with decreased cognitive abilities. In one study, men who ate a diet rich in folate had decreased levels of homocysteine and, as a result, their memories were better protected.

OTHER AREAS OF IMPORTANCE IN NUTRITION

Water. As you grow older, drinking plenty of water is vital. Aging can cause your ability to detect thirst to decrease; therefore, drink water even when you are not thirsty. Being dehydrated can create a higher potency of medication in the body, an important fact for people who take high doses of medications. Finally, dehydration can have a negative impact on mental performance. In fact, a mere 2% dip in hydration level can cause a 7% decrease in short-term memory and a 13% decrease in concentration.

Supplements. There are many claims that certain vitamin supplements can improve memory. You may even have seen magic pills that claim to prevent Alzheimer's disease. No supplement, however, has been proven to have a consistent and reliable impact on memory. If there are supplements that you are currently taking or would like to try, make sure to speak with your doctor first and tell him or her about all other medications that you are taking. It can be dangerous to mix some vitamins and herbs with over-the-counter or prescription medication. One supplement that is generally considered safe and important for older adults is a multivitamin that contains the B vitamins, which, as mentioned earlier, are important for maintaining memory. Also, as you grow older, your ability to absorb these vitamins from foods decreases.

Curry. Studies have shown that curry or, more specifically, curcumin, a spice used in making turmeric (a popular ingredient in curry), may have brain-protecting benefits. Curcumin is a powerful antioxidant and has anti-inflammatory properties that may enhance memory. Some research shows that South Asian and Indian nations, who are among the highest users of the spice, have lower rates of Alzheimer's disease (*Daily Mail Reporter*, 2008).

Coffee. For women who enjoy a cup of coffee (or more) a day, there is encouraging research that shows the beneficial effects of coffee on memory. A 2007 French study found that women age 65 and older who drank three or more cups of coffee each day performed higher on tests that measured thinking and memory skills (Ritchie et al., 2007). Researchers also found, however, that the same protective benefits do not extend to men, perhaps because men metabolize coffee differently or because women may be more sensitive to the effects of caffeine.

EAT MORE HEALTHY FOODS

There is always room to boost the level of nutritious, brain-healthy foods in your diet, and doing so isn't as hard as it may seem. Experts recommend a minimum of five servings of fruits and vegetables every day. How might you fit it all in? Eat half a cup of strawberries with breakfast, fill your sandwich with veggies for lunch, and have broccoli or salad with dinner. Then make sure that you eat at least two snacks during the day (apple slices, carrot sticks, a banana). You'll be surprised how quickly you reach your five servings.

Another way to make sure that you are eating plenty of healthy foods it to "eat the rainbow." This means to make sure that you eat at least one food of every color each day—red apples, orange peppers, yellow pineapple, green spinach, blueberries, and purple grapes. Mix it up, and try new fruits and vegetables, too!

Nutrition
FACILITATOR INSTRUCTIONS

1. WELCOME AND INTRODUCTION (10 MINUTES)

To do before class:

- Read and familiarize yourself with the Nutrition Overview.

- Write the following quote on a board or flip chart.

> "Vegetables are a must on a diet. I suggest
> carrot cake, zucchini bread, and pumpkin pie."
> (Garfield, from cartoonist Jim Davis)

- Familiarize yourself with and make appropriate copies of the warm-up activity, quiz, practice activities, and homework.

Greet the participants and make introductions, if necessary. Explain that the class will focus on nutrition and its effect on memory. Ask participants to think about what they ate yesterday for breakfast, lunch, and dinner (or today, if the class is in the evening). Ask them to keep their answers in the back of their minds until later for a class discussion. Explain that today we know more about nutrition and its effect on memory than ever before, and that research shows eating the right foods can help to improve memory. The good news is that most of the recommended foods actually taste good, too. (Doughnuts, however, are not on the list!)

Discuss the quote and ask participants for their interpretations. Ask how many of them actually enjoy vegetables in their diet.

2. WARM-UP ACTIVITY (10 MINUTES)

Pass out the worksheet *Name 10 Foods that Are Yellow* and explain that the activity will help get participants' minds warmed up to learn about nutrition. In addition, it's an excellent brain-boosting activity because it will force participants to use their brains in ways that they might not have otherwise. Encourage them to list all of the foods that they can think of, even if they come up with more than 10.

3.   QUIZ (15 MINUTES)

There are many myths and false beliefs about which foods are good for the body and the brain. Distribute the *Nutrition and Memory Quiz* and give participants about 5 minutes to complete it. Remind everyone that it is all right if they don't know all of the answers and to do the best they can. After everyone has finished, review each answer, pausing for questions and comments as you go along. Ask participants how they did and explain that they will learn more during class about the areas of nutrition discussed in the quiz.

4.   EXPLANATION AND DISCUSSION OF NUTRITION AND HOW IT AFFECTS MEMORY (25 MINUTES)

Review the facilitator overview located at the beginning of the lesson. Discuss the importance of antioxidants, omega-3 fatty acids, and dark green, leafy vegetables. Write each of the three categories on a board or flip chart and ask participants to give examples of foods that fit in each category. Finally, discuss the other important areas of nutrition (water, supplements, curry, and coffee), as well as ways to eat more brain-healthy foods.

5.   PRACTICE ACTIVITIES (20 MINUTES)

After discussing which foods are high in antioxidants, distribute the handout *Foods High in Antioxidants* and ask participants to review it. Ask them to name some foods from the list that they eat regularly. Then ask them to choose at least one food that they have never tried or don't eat regularly and encourage them to try it this week!

Next, review and discuss the section "Other Areas of Importance in Nutrition," pausing for questions and comments.

Distribute the table *Nutrition and Memory* and explain that it offers a good overview of brain-healthy foods and dietary habits. Encourage participants to keep the table someplace where they will see it every day. Tell them that it is a wonderful tool to use when making a grocery list!

Ask participants if they feel they eat as nutritiously as possible all of the time. Explain that it can be hard to fit all of the recommended nutritious foods into their diet every day, but that there are some tips that can make it easier for them to do so (review the section "Eat More Healthy Foods").

Explain to the group that now that they have a good idea of which foods are brain healthy and how to incorporate more of these foods into their daily diet, they next will practice turning a meal of their choice into a super brain-healthy meal. Pass out the worksheet *Make Over Your Meal* and ask participants to choose at least one meal to make more brain healthy. Give them about 5 minutes to complete the activity and encourage them, if they would like, to choose more than one meal to make healthier. After everyone has finished, ask for volunteers to share their makeover ideas.

6.   REVIEW AND CLOSING (5 MINUTES)

Thank the group for their participation and encourage them to try as least one healthy new food this week. Review the importance of antioxidants, omega-3 fatty acids, and dark green, leafy vegetables. Remind participants that although it is impossible to eat brain-healthy foods 100% of the time, every effort counts toward better nutrition and improved mental alertness. Ask if anyone has any final questions.

7.   HOMEWORK (5 MINUTES)

Pass out the homework sheets and explain what should be done for each. Encourage everyone to complete them during the week. Remind them that homework should be fun and to enlist the help of family and friends, if they can.

- *Vegetable Word Scramble*

- *Indian, Italian, French, and Other Regional Foods*

- Practice incorporating more fruits and veggies into your daily diet!

Nutrition
CLASS AGENDA

1. Welcome and Introduction
2. Warm-Up Activity
   - *Name 10 Foods that Are Yellow*
3. Quiz
   - *Nutrition and Memory Quiz*
4. Overview of Nutrition and How It Affects Memory
   - Antioxidants
   - Omega-3 Fatty Acids
   - Dark Green, Leafy Vegetables
5. Practice Activities
   - *Foods High in Antioxidants*
   - *Nutrition and Memory*
   - *Make Over Your Meal*
6. Review and Closing
7. Homework
   - *Vegetable Word Scramble*
   - *Indian, Italian, French, and Other Regional Foods*
   - Practice incorporating more vegetables and fruits into your diet!

Strengthen Your Mind Program: A Course for Memory Enhancement by Einberger & Sellick.

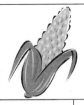

Name 10 Foods that Are Yellow

List at least 10 foods that are commonly yellow.

1.

2.

3.

4.

5.

6.

7.

8.

9.

10.

Strengthen Your Mind Program: A Course for Memory Enhancement by Einberger & Sellick.

171

Nutrition and Memory Quiz

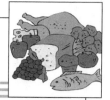

The following questions will test your knowledge of healthy foods. Circle your answers.

1. Which of the following has more vitamins and nutrients?
   A. red pepper
   B. green pepper

2. True or False: As you grow older and less active you need fewer nutrients in your diet.

3. Which of the following foods has the most Vitamin B_{12}?
   A. potato
   B. snapper
   C. chocolate chip cookie
   D. squash

4. Which meal is the least brain healthy?
   A. turkey, iceberg lettuce salad, mashed potatoes
   B. salmon, wild rice salad, broccoli
   C. hamburger, french fries, green grapes

5. Which is higher in antioxidants?
   A. pink grapefruit
   B. white grapefruit
   C. neither of the above

6. Which type of chocolate is better for you?
   A. dark
   B. milk
   C. white

7. Which of the following is not a good source of omega-3 fatty acids?
   A. walnuts
   B. salmon
   C. flaxseeds
   D. peanuts

8. True or False: If you have problems with urinary incontinence, you should cut back on your water intake.

9. Staying hydrated is especially important for older adults. Which of the following does not count toward daily liquid intake?
   A. tea or coffee
   B. reduced sodium soup
   C. martini
   D. nonfat milk

Strengthen Your Mind Program: A Course for Memory Enhancement by Einberger & Sellick.

Nutrition and Memory Quiz ANSWER SHEET

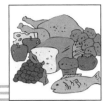

1. **Which of the following has more vitamins and nutrients?**

   A. *red pepper*. Foods that are brighter in color are more nutritionally dense and contain more antioxidants.

2. **True or False: As you grow older and less active you need fewer nutrients in your diet.**

   False. As you grow older you may need fewer calories to maintain your weight. It is important, however, to maintain a diet rich in nutrients, which means eating foods that give you the most "nutritional bang for the buck."

3. **Which of the following foods has the most Vitamin B_{12}?**

   B. *snapper*. B_{12} vitamins are found in most animal products. Especially good sources include lean beef, liver, dairy, and some seafood.

4. **Which meal is the least brain healthy?**

   C. *hamburger, french fries, green grapes*. Unless the hamburger is loaded with vegetables, there is not much nutrition to be found in this meal. French fries are laden with calories and have almost no nutritional content. The green grapes offer some nutrients, but red grapes contain more brain-healthy antioxidants.

5. **Which is higher in antioxidants?**

   A. *pink grapefruit*. The darker colored grapefruit contains more antioxidants.

6. **Which type of chocolate is better for you?**

   A. *dark*. Dark chocolate contains flavanoids, a powerful antioxidant. White chocolate is actually not a chocolate (it contains no cocoa at all).

7. **Which of the following is not a good source of omega-3 fatty acids?**

   D. *peanuts*. The best source of omega-3 fatty acids is fish, such as salmon, mackerel, and sardines. Walnuts, flaxseeds, canola oil, and some fortified eggs are also good sources.

8. **True or False: If you have problems with urinary incontinence, you should cut back on your water intake.**

   False. Even if you have problems with incontinence or if you are taking medications that cause you to urinate frequently, you still need to drink enough water each day. Experts recommend at least six glasses of liquid each day, and water is the healthiest liquid that you can drink.

9. **Staying hydrated is especially important for older adults. Which of the following does not count toward daily liquid intake?**

   C. *martini*. Alcohol is a diuretic that actually makes your lose water and can contribute to dehydration. Caffeine is also a diuretic. If you drink caffeinated tea, coffee, or other liquids, be sure to do so in moderation, or drink decaffeinated versions instead. If you have bladder problems or incontinence, you should avoid foods and liquids that contain caffeine.

Foods High in Antioxidants

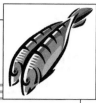

Antioxidants have received the most attention of all the dietary factors that are being investigated for possible roles in staving off mental decline with aging. Red and orange fruits and vegetables and most dark green vegetables are particularly high in antioxidants. The following foods are among the most rich in antioxidants.

kale

spinach

Brussels sprouts

prunes

raisins

blueberries

blackberries

broccoli

beets

red bell peppers

eggplant

oranges

strawberries

raspberries

plums

almonds, pecans, walnuts

red leaf lettuce

red apples

red kidney beans

red cabbage

carrots

tomatoes

yams

whole grains

(And, of course, dark chocolate!)

 Strengthen Your Mind Program: A Course for Memory Enhancement by Einberger & Sellick.
© 2010 by Health Professions Press, Inc.

Nutrition and Memory

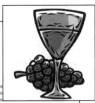

The following foods can help keep your memory sharp.

	Benefits	Examples
B vitamins (B_6, B_{12}, and folic acid)	• Protect brain nerve cells from homocysteine, high levels of which have been associated with decreased cognitive abilities. • Critical to keeping memory sharp. • Associated with faster processing of information and memory recall.	• Spinach • Dark, leafy greens • Asparagus • Broccoli • Strawberries • Melons • Black beans, soybeans, and other legumes • Citrus fruits
Antioxidants	• Protect cells from damage caused by free radicals. • Reduce cell oxidation, which may contribute to aging and cognitive decline. • Help to improve blood flow to the brain.	• Fruits and vegetables (see *Foods High in Antioxidants*).
Breakfast	• People who eat breakfast score higher on memory tests and report better mood.	• Combine a high-protein food with a high-fiber starch (e.g., eggs and whole wheat toast).
Omega-3 fatty acids	• May prevent memory decline. • Decrease the risk of developing dementia.	• Salmon • Mackerel • Lake trout • Herring • Sardines • Albacore tuna • Flaxseeds • Canola and soybean oils • Walnuts
Hydration	• Even mild dehydration can cause confusion and have a negative impact on mental performance and concentration.	• Water is best • Decaffeinated tea, coffee, or soda • Soups • Fruits • Vegetables
Curry, red wine, and dark chocolate	• Curry has been shown to protect brain cells. • Red wine and chocolate contain flavanoids, which can help to reduce the risk of dementia by preventing the breakdown of brain cells.	• South Asian and Indian foods • Pinot Noir, Cabernet Sauvignon, and Petit Syrah • Dark chocolate has far more flavanoids than milk chocolate or white chocolate

Make Over Your Meal

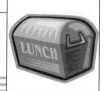

Take a few minutes to think about how you can improve your nutrition. Take a mental inventory of what you eat every day, including snacks and drinks. Choose at least one meal and make it over to include as many brain-healthy foods as possible.

Meal: Breakfast
  What I usually eat _____

  _____

  How can I improve? _____

  _____

Meal: Lunch
  What I usually eat _____

  _____

  How can I improve? _____

  _____

Meal: Dinner
  What I usually eat _____

  _____

  How can I improve? _____

  _____

Snacks
  What I usually eat _____

  _____

  How can I improve? _____

  _____

Vegetable Word Scramble

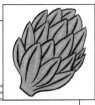

Unscramble the following words to reveal a delicious, brain-healthy vegetable!

buccremu _____

pgasraasu _____

rotcsra _____

cwoflirauel _____

noRieam tceuelt _____

mosomhusr _____

ngtelpag _____

uslesrBs opsstru _____

iuzhicnc _____

cinhpas _____

innoo _____

lelb preppe _____

rnoc _____

motaot _____

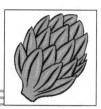

buccremu	**cucumber**
pgasraasu	**asparagus**
rotcsra	**carrots**
cwoflirauel	**cauliflower**
noRieam tceuelt	**Romaine lettuce**
mosomhusr	**mushrooms**
ngtelpag	**eggplant**
uslesrBs opsstru	**Brussels sprouts**
iuzhicnc	**zucchini**
cinhpas	**spinach**
innoo	**onion**
lelb preppe	**bell pepper**
rnoc	**corn**
motaot	**tomato**

Strengthen Your Mind Program: A Course for Memory Enhancement by Einberger & Sellick.
© 2010 by Health Professions Press, Inc.

Indian, Italian, French, and Other Regional Foods

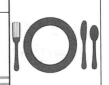

More and more, ethnic foods are found in stores, in restaurants, and at the dinner tables of friends. "American" food is expanding! Each of the following foods is particularly associated with a state, area, or foreign country. Can you name these places?

1. Yorkshire pudding (popover-like bread served with roast beef)

2. Gelato (dense, rich ice cream)

3. Hummus (mixture containing mashed chickpeas)

4. Ratatouille (vegetable stew)

5. Poi (fermented paste made from taro root)

6. Sushi (raw fish and rice wrapped in seaweed)

7. Chai (sweet, spiced tea)

8. Paella (rice dish with meat, seafood, and vegetables)

9. Chianti (dry, red wine)

10. Crepes (thin pancakes)

11. Sauerbraten (marinated beef cooked with vinegar)

12. Baklava (sweet pastry of phyllo dough, nuts, spice, and honey-lemon syrup)

13. Escargot (edible snails)

14. Chutney (relish made from fruit, spices, and herbs)

15. Grits (coarsely ground corn)

16. Goulash (stew seasoned with paprika)

17. Tamales (meat filling wrapped in cornhusks)

18. Tapas (small appetizers)

19. Schnitzel (fried veal cutlet)

20. Sake (wine made from rice)

Indian, Italian, French, and Other Regional Foods ANSWER SHEET

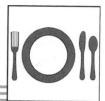

1. Yorkshire pudding   **England**

2. Gelato   **Italy**

3. Hummus   **Middle East**

4. Ratatouille   **France**

5. Poi   **Hawaii**

6. Sushi   **Japan**

7. Chai   **India**

8. Paella   **Spain**

9. Chianti   **Italy**

10. Crepes   **France**

11. Sauerbraten   **Germany**

12. Baklava   **Greece/Turkey**

13. Escargot   **France**

14. Chutney   **India**

15. Grits   **Southern United States**

16. Goulash   **Hungary**

17. Tamales   **Mexico**

18. Tapas   **Spain**

19. Schnitzel   **Austria**

20. Sake   **Japan**

Socialization

Socialization
FACILITATOR OVERVIEW

Socializing with friends, family, and new acquaintances has multiple benefits—it is fun, reduces stress, makes us feel needed, is good for our bodies, and, as we now know, is good for our brains. This class, as with all of the others, should be experiential; the very nature of the subject dictates that it be so. Leave plenty of time for spontaneous socialization and fun. Be sure that everyone is included and that no one is isolated.

SOCIAL INTEGRATION VERSUS MENTAL DECLINE

Increasing evidence shows that people who are socially active live longer and remain more independent than those who are isolated. A study on socialization conducted by Ertel, Glymour, and Berkman (2008) of the Harvard School of Public Health analyzed data gathered from 1998 to 2004 as part of a large study on health and retirement in the United States involving a nationally representative population of adults age 50 and older. Memory was assessed at 2-year intervals. Social integration was assessed by marital status, volunteer activities, and contact with parents, children, and neighbors. Results showed that individuals with the highest social integration had the slowest rate of memory decline from 1998 to 2004, and memory decline among the most integrated was less than half the rate among the least integrated. The researchers concluded that:

> Social participation and integration have profound effects on health and well-being of people during their lifetimes. We know from previous studies that people with many social ties have lower mortality rates. We now have mounting evidence that strong social networks can help to prevent declines in memory. As our society ages and has more and more older people, it will be important to promote their engagement in social and community life to maintain their well-being.

A 5-year study by the Kaiser Permanente Southern California Department of Research and Evaluation, funded by the National Institute on Aging, found that a strong social network of family and friends is associated with a lower risk of dementia (Crooks et al., 2008). The researchers followed 2,249 women age 78 and older who had not been diagnosed with dementia. Those with large social networks were roughly 26% less likely to develop dementia when compared to women with smaller social networks. The researchers suggested that a possible reason for the findings could be that social networks facilitate healthy behaviors, such as joining a walking group, tennis team, or bowling league. Dr. Richard Della Penna, medical director of the Kaiser Permanente Aging Network, summarized the findings as follows:

> This well-done study significantly adds to the growing body of information that lifestyle, cognitive activity, and social connectivity appear to reduce the risk of dementia and help maintain a healthy brain, and my advice to older adults is to maintain and even increase their social ties.

Another study conducted by David Bennett, M.D., and his colleagues was the first to examine the relationship between social networks and the symptoms of Alzheimer's disease (Rush University Medical Center, 2006). The study involved people whose brains had large numbers of plaques and tangles—the hallmarks of Alzheimer's disease. Some developed traditional symptoms of the disease, such as memory loss and dementia, while others did not. The difference between the two was that for those people with larger social networks, the changes of Alzheimer's were much less likely to result in memory loss than for those with smaller social networks. Thus, despite the fact that the brains of everyone involved in the study had the tangles and plaques indicative of Alzheimer's disease, those with larger social networks appear to have been protected from the damaging effects of the disease (Rush University Medical Center, 2006).

INCREASING SOCIAL OUTLETS

In general, many other studies show the same results as those discussed in this overview, and more are currently being conducted. Socializing is indeed good for brain health. The opposite is also true—isolation and loneliness are bad for the brain and can take years off of someone's life. Strong social contacts have the power to protect a person against the mental decline that often goes along with aging. As we age, maintaining these contacts is increasingly important. The more we socialize, the more we are able to keep our minds sharp. We must make socialization an integral and continual part of our lives. We need to find ways to foster friendships, to maintain family ties, to make new friends, to try new things, to volunteer, and to be passionate about life.

Socializing is a great mental exercise and can be done in a number of different ways. How can we stay socially connected as we age? The handout *Expanding Your Social Horizon* lists many activities. Encourage participants, however, not to be limited by the list (they will be asked to add other activities that are of interest to them). When we open our minds, new possibilities avail themselves to us!

Socialization
FACILITATOR INSTRUCTIONS

1. WELCOME AND INTRODUCTION (10 MINUTES)

To do before class:

- Read and familiarize yourself with the Socialization Overview.

- Write the following quotes on a board or flip chart:

> We cannot live only for ourselves. A thousand fibers connect us with
> our fellow men.
> (Herman Melville, novelist)

> No man is an island, entire of itself; every man is a piece of the continent,
> a part of the main.
> (John Donne, poet)

> Shared joy is a double joy; shared sorrow is half a sorrow.
> (Swedish proverb)

- Familiarize yourself with and make appropriate copies of the warm-up activity, quiz, practice activities, and homework.

Welcome participants and make introductions, if necessary. Explain that the focus of the class will be socialization and its effect on memory. Ask how many of the participants consider themselves to be fairly social. Do they believe that their level of social connectedness has an effect on their memory? Tell them that they will learn the answer to this important question as part of the class.

Discuss the three quotes and ask participants for their interpretations.

2. WARM-UP ACTIVITY (GROUP ACTIVITY) (10 MINUTES)

Ask everyone to choose a partner. Have each of the partners spend 5 minutes talking to each other and coming up with 5 things that they have in common. This could be hair color or favorite food, place to eat, actor, hobby, sports figure, and so forth. Encourage the partners to explore a wide range of ideas. This is a great way to get people involved with each other to begin the class. Ask for volunteers to share what they have in common with their partner.

3. QUIZ (10 MINUTES)

People often don't think about the importance of leading an active social life. Ask participants to complete the questionnaire *How Social Are You?* Explain that this activity will give them the opportunity to review their social outlets and identify areas where it may be good for them to make improvements. After participants complete the questionnaire, ask if they are happy with their answers. If not, challenge them to think of ways that they might increase certain aspects of their social life.

4. EXPLANATION AND DISCUSSION OF SOCIALIZATION AND HOW IT AFFECTS MEMORY (25 MINUTES)

Discuss with the class the research presented in the overview on socialization and its effects on the brain and memory. Ask participants to list other possible benefits of socialization. What are some of the negative effects of leading an isolated life? Distribute the handout *Expanding Your Social Horizon*. Review the list and encourage participants to add to it activities that are of interest to them.

5. PRACTICE ACTIVITIES (25 MINUTES)

Pass out the worksheet *Volunteering*. Give participants 5 minutes to complete it. Suggest that they consider volunteering in some way, if they are not already doing so, noting the many benefits. Encourage them to think of other possible opportunities for volunteering. Ask participants to share with the class their own experiences volunteering.

A perfect way to reinforce the importance of an active social life is to have the class get up, move about the room, and converse with other members of the group. Pass out *Get to Know Your Classmates* and give participants 10 minutes to find a different person for each characteristic. If the group is large enough, there should be one person for each characteristic. If the group is small, allow two characteristics per person. After the group has completed the activity, suggest that participants may want to do the same activity in a group to which they belong, possibly changing some of the characteristics to better suit the particular group. Examples may be:

- Find someone whose favorite baseball team is the same as yours or whose golf handicap is similar to yours for a sports groups.

- Find someone who loves to cook with lots of fresh herbs for a cooking group.

- Find someone whose favorite card game is the same as yours for a game group.

This activity is a great icebreaker when people in the group don't know each other.

6. REVIEW AND CLOSING (5 MINUTES)

Thank the group for their participation. Express that hopefully the socialization that took place in the class will spur participants to expand their social horizons. Note how enjoyable it was to teach the class and that hopefully the group had fun socializing with their classmates. Encourage participants to increase their level of socialization and to keep in mind the important benefits of doing so.

7.   HOMEWORK (5 MINUTES)

Pass out the homework sheets and explain what should be done for each. Stress the importance of completing the assignments; they will help remind participants of the importance of maintaining and expanding their social lives.

- *Expanding Your Social Life*

- *In the Neighborhood*

- Call, write, or get together with a friend you haven't been in touch with in quite some time.

Socialization
CLASS AGENDA

1. Welcome and Introduction
2. Warm-Up Activity
   - Commonalities (Group Activity)
3. Quiz
   - *How Social Are You?*
4. Overview of Socialization and How It Affects Memory
   - *Expanding Your Social Horizon*
5. Practice Activities
   - *Volunteering*
   - *Get to Know Your Classmates*
6. Review and Closing
7. Homework
   - *Expanding Your Social Life*
   - *In the Neighborhood*
   - Call, write, or get together with a friend you haven't been in touch with in quite some time.

How Social Are You?

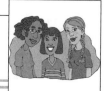

Answer yes or no to the following questions to give you an idea of how active your social life is and how involved you are in your community.

1. I talk to/see my friends on a regular basis.

2. I talk to/see family on a regular basis.

3. I sometimes create opportunities to speak with my neighbors, such as when getting the mail or walking the dog.

4. I belong to at least one community group (church, club, choir, service group).

5. I regularly visit places where I have the opportunity to converse with others (library, farmers' market, coffee house).

6. I currently volunteer in some capacity or have done so in the last few months.

7. I have at least one good friend with whom I get together on a regular basis.

8. I take advantage of new learning opportunities in my community (attending classes, lectures, and/or special presentations).

9. I attend local events (plays, the symphony, art exhibit, bingo night, crafts fair, holiday shows).

10. I take advantage of opportunities to engage in physical activities with others (walking, bocce ball, bowling, exercise class).

11. I get together with friends and/or family to engage in mind-stimulating activities (play board games or cards, read, cook).

12. I value friendships and enjoy the company of others.

Strengthen Your Mind Program: A Course for Memory Enhancement by Einberger & Sellick.

Expanding Your Social Horizon

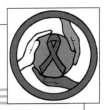

The following is a list of groups, classes, clubs, and activities that may interest you as you expand your social horizon. Add your own ideas to the list. Be sure to surround yourself with positive people when you engage in any activity! From the list pick one activity that you are not currently involved in and give it a try over the next couple of months. Or try an activity not listed here. Remember, not only is being socially involved a great way to enhance your memory, but also to reduce some of the stress that somehow manages to creep into our lives!

Sports leagues

Support groups

Church activities

Adult education courses

Art classes

Health clubs

Pet shows

Photography classes or clubs

Golf or other group sports

Alumni groups

Dance classes

Language classes

Biking clubs

Wine-tasting clubs or classes

Book clubs

Singles/widows/widower groups

Card clubs

Scrabble clubs

Collectors clubs (stamps, coins)

Computer groups or classes

College courses

Drama groups

Choir groups

Outdoor clubs (hiking, canoeing, bird-watching)

Volunteering

Museum groups

Social or political activities

Environmental activism

Writing groups

Community gardens

Professional organizations

Travel groups

Volunteering

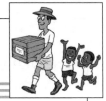

The benefits of volunteering, of doing good things for others, are many. It is good not only for those for whom we are volunteering and for the community at large, but also for ourselves. Among the personal benefits are decreased stress, depression, loneliness, and isolation as well as an increased sense of self-worth, improved health, and better brain fitness. As we age these benefits become more important than ever in helping us to maintain and enhance memory.

Consider volunteer opportunities in your community, such as those through a food bank, the library, the local museum, schools, government, political parties, hospitals, and a host of other possibilities. Contact a volunteer agency, look for volunteer listings in the local newspaper, or talk to others—all have the potential to open up new ideas.

Below, list some possible volunteer opportunities for yourself and then brainstorm next steps to make the possibilities into realities.

Strengthen Your Mind Program: A Course for Memory Enhancement by Einberger & Sellick.

Get to Know Your Classmates

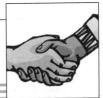

Find a person in the class with whom you share in common the following. You need to find a different person for each list entry.

1. Favorite color.

2. Favorite season.

3. Has traveled outside of the United States.

4. Was in the Armed Forces.

5. Was born in the same area of the United States as you.

6. Favorite type of music.

7. Favorite comedian.

8. Exercises at least four times a week.

9. Speaks a language other than English.

10 Favorite baseball or football team.

11. Favorite ice cream flavor.

12. Favorite holiday.

13. Has the same color eyes as you.

14. Has the same number of children as you.

15. Whose name has the same number of syllables as yours.

16. Favorite candy bar.

17. Favorite type of reading material.

18. Loves to travel just about anywhere, anytime.

Strengthen Your Mind Program: A Course for Memory Enhancement by Einberger & Sellick.
© 2010 by Health Professions Press, Inc.

Expanding Your Social Life

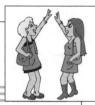

Review the list *Expanding Your Social Horizon*. Now that you've learned the many benefits of a full social life, especially for your brain, pick from the list three ways to try to expand your social life that you'll focus on in the coming weeks. How can you make them happen? Do you need to make some calls, look for listings in the local newspaper, or visit the library or senior center? Whatever you decide to try, list the steps you need to take and begin the journey!

1.

2.

3.

Strengthen Your Mind Program: A Course for Memory Enhancement by Einberger & Sellick.

In the Neighborhood

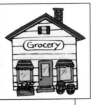

Neighborhoods vary from urban to farm, and suburban to rural; however, each type of neighborhood has a life of its own. Regardless of the type(s) of neighborhood you grew up in, most have a variety of fun, games, and social opportunities. Read the following descriptions of neighborhood life. Can you name each item?

1.   These large round hoops are popular with kids, who swing them around their hips for fun.

2.   This bill given to veterans by the military helped fund the boom in suburban housing in the 1950s.

3.   Kids made these ride-on toys or "bugs" out of old apple boxes attached to roller skate wheels.

4.   Kids could often be found outside playing this game, which consisted of one person designated as "it," other kids hiding, and a can.

5.   These types of parties generally involve the whole neighborhood and can be held for holidays or other celebrations.

6.   This type of socializing involved teenagers driving around town, often on a particular street to see friends.

7.   Similar to an ice cream parlor, this type of establishment served colas, malts, and milkshakes.

8.   Many children in the neighborhood joined clubs for social and educational opportunities. Try to list at least three.

9.   After dinner most families would gather around this electronic device, which most households had by the end of the 1950s.

10.   This person was a staple in the neighborhood and delivered milk and other dairy products to the doorstep of homes.

11.   This type of party made it possible to purchase popular plastic storage containers and provided an opportunity for women to socialize and meet new friends.

12.   This truck had an attention-grabbing musical jingle and generally drove around after dinner.

13.   This common children's game is usually played on the sidewalk and involves drawing a series of squares on which players have to jump.

14.   With this type of dinner party you travel from house to house, meeting neighbors while enjoying a different dinner course at each location.

15.   This television show was popular with kids in the 1970s, '80s, and '90s and featured a musical host who began each show with the song "Won't you be my neighbor?"

16.   In this form of fundraising, a person (usually a woman) makes a lunch that is "auctioned" to the highest bidder, who traditionally then has a date with or shares lunch with the woman who made it.

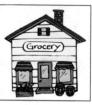

1. These large round hoops are popular with kids, who swing them around their hips for fun.
    hula hoop

2. This bill given to veterans by the military helped fund the boom in suburban housing in the 1950s.
    GI Bill

3. Kids made this ride-on toy or "bug" out of an old apple box attached to roller skate wheels.
    soapbox car

4. Kids could often be found outside playing this game, which consisted of one person designated as "it," other kids hiding, and a can.
    kick the can

5. These types of parties generally involve the whole neighborhood and can be held for holidays or other celebrations.
    block party

6. This type of socializing involved teenagers driving around town, often on a particular street to see friends.
    cruising

7. Similar to an ice cream parlor, this type of establishment served colas, malts, and milkshakes.
    soda shop

8. Many children in the neighborhood joined clubs for social and educational opportunities. Try to list at least three.
    Boy Scouts, Girl Scouts, 4-H, Campfire Girls

9. After dinner most families would gather around this electronic device, which most households had by the end of the 1950s.
    television

10. This person was a staple in the neighborhood and delivered milk and other dairy products to the doorstep of homes.
    milkman

11. This type of party made it possible to purchase popular plastic storage containers and provided an opportunity for women to socialize and meet new friends.
    Tupperware party

12. This truck had an attention-grabbing musical jingle and generally drove around after dinner.
    ice cream truck

13. This common children's game is usually played on the sidewalk and involves drawing a series of squares on which players have to jump.
    hopscotch

14. With this type of dinner party you travel from house to house, meeting neighbors while enjoying a different dinner course at each location.
    progressive dinner party

15. This television show was popular with kids in the 1970s, '80s, and '90s and featured a musical host who began each show with the song "Won't you be my neighbor?"
    Mister Rogers' Neighborhood

16. In this form of fundraising, a person (usually a woman) makes a lunch that is "auctioned" to the highest bidder, who traditionally then has a date with or shares lunch with the woman who made it.
    box social

Memory-Enhancement Course Review

Memory-Enhancement Course Review
FACILITATOR OVERVIEW

Memory can be enhanced in many ways. Each of the 11 classes has given participants the opportunity to learn new information in a variety of ways, all of which help to ensure that new information will be remembered. The class topics are those that the authors believe are among the most important for memory enhancement. Research continues in each of the areas covered in the classes and additional ways to learn new information and improve memory are continually discovered. Encourage participants always to search for techniques to improve their memory, to stay active, and to learn new things.

The following sections are a brief overview of each class.

MEMORY AND AGING

Contrary to what many people believe, memory loss is not an inevitable part of aging. Whereas it was commonly thought that "you can't teach an old dog new tricks," we now know that even as people grow older they are able to learn and challenge their brains. There are some changes in memory, however, that are to be expected: it takes longer to process new information and to recall information, and it becomes more difficult to multi-task or pay attention to more than one thing at a time.

A person continues to grow new neurons, or nerve cells, throughout life, a process called neurogenesis. This ability to grow new nerve cells is what allows and supports brain plasticity, which is the brain's capacity to learn and remember new information in response to influences and experiences as a person ages. Although it is true that we lose thousands of brain cells each day, new ones can be created, which means that the brain is able to learn new information, create new ideas, and, most important, change in response to learning as a person ages. Suggestions throughout the class on Memory and Aging will hopefully have helped participants to use a variety of different techniques to both learn new information and remember what they have learned. You can, indeed, teach an old dog new tricks, but it takes practice, practice, practice!

LEARNING STYLES

Learning styles are different ways in which people process information in order to be able to learn it and apply it. There are three basic learning styles: auditory, visual, and tactile/kinesthetic. Auditory learners need to hear and process new information out loud or to themselves. Visual learners need to see or read information or take notes. Tactile/kinesthetic learners need to touch and feel things and prefer hands-on learning.

We learn using all three learning styles; however, most of us tend to prefer one style more than the other two and learn best in that way. It's important for us to learn how best to use our dominant learning style most efficiently for optimum memory, but it's also important to practice using the other two styles to give us more tools with which to learn.

MENTAL AEROBICS

As one ages it is important to exercise the brain to keep memory sharp. There are many brain-stimulating, or mental aerobic, activities to do, including working on word puzzles, reading, being creative (painting, taking photographs), playing games, learning a new language, taking a class, and becoming involved in the creative arts. Music is one of the most powerful tools to enhance memory, and it is important to incorporate more of it into everyday life (listening to music, learning an instrument, singing).

To stimulate the brain in new and different ways you need to try new activities as well as vary the way you do some of your daily activities. Stimulating your brain in new and different ways is what causes new nerve cells to grow, which is the hallmark of the brain's ability to change and grow in response to learning (brain plasticity).

EXERCISE

The three main types of exercise (cardiovascular, strength training, and stretching and flexibility) when done in moderation can benefit the body and mind. Each has a variety of benefits, including lowering heart rate and blood pressure, speeding up metabolism, strengthening muscles, improving balance and coordination, and increasing range of motion in the joints. All three types of exercise can be done with little or no equipment.

Exercise, when done on a regular basis, can also improve cognitive functioning, increase the ability to multitask, improve recall, and may help to slow the progression of memory-related illnesses. One of the main reasons for these benefits is that exercise helps maintain blood flow to the brain as people age, and better blood flow translates into improved cognition.

Getting into the habit of exercising takes some practice, but little steps can add up to big results. When a person does exercise, he or she generally feels better all over. It's important to find types of exercise that you enjoy and get moving!

STRATEGIES FOR MEMORY IMPROVEMENT

There are many strategies for improving memory, including paying careful attention (focusing and limiting multitasking); visualization (taking a picture of something in your mind's eye and using that image to help remember the item); and chunking (breaking down large pieces of information into smaller chunks of information that are easier to retain in short-term memory). Other strategies include mnemonics (a phrase that helps you to remember a list or specific information); association (linking an item to be remembered with something that you already know); repetition (repeating information to yourself to remember it); creating a story to link bits of information together; and creating a visual reminder (physically moving an item so that it is out of place and more likely to catch your eye). It is important to learn which strategies are most effective for you and to incorporate them into your everyday life.

BRAIN DOMINANCE

There are two sides of the brain—the right side, which is the more creative, unpredictable, philosophical, visual, intuitive, and active part of the brain, and the left side, which is more analytical, sequential, organized, and verbal.

People use the right and left sides of the brain to process different kinds of information. For the most part, people use one side of their brain more often and more efficiently than the other in thinking and learning. It is important, however, that a person become more whole-brained by learning to use both sides of the brain efficiently. The more efficiently both sides of the brain are used, the more brain power a person has to enhance memory!

THE FIVE SENSES

There are five basic senses—sight, hearing, touch, taste, and smell. Everything we know and everything we learn comes to us through our senses. Our vision is responsible for taking in the greatest amount of information, followed by our hearing. Most experts agree, however, that it is our sense of smell that triggers memories more than any of the other four senses, memories that can last an extremely long time, even a lifetime.

Generally the senses decline with age. Through practice, however, we can learn to use all of our senses more fully, even as we grow older. The more consciously we use all of our senses, the more information we collect and the easier that information is to recall. In other words, the more information we receive through a variety of paths, the more likely we are to remember the information. If we truly use all of our senses in combination with one another, we stand the greatest likelihood of being able to enhance our memories.

STRESS

Too much stress adversely affects the body by raising blood pressure and resting heart rate, lowering immunity, and generally worsening overall health. Too much stress can also affect mental and emotional health by increasing the likelihood of depression, decreasing the ability to focus, and making it difficult to deal with the decisions and routines of everyday life.

Research has shown that stress can also take a toll on the brain and memory. Too much stress causes the brain to release stress hormones that adversely affect memory. The main culprit is the stress hormone called cortisol, too much of which can prevent the brain from forming a new memory or from recalling an existing memory.

We all experience stress in our everyday lives. It is important that we learn to manage stress and not allow it to affect memory. There are a number of stress-management techniques that we need to take the time to practice on a regular basis to keep the body and mind healthy.

OPTIMISM AND HUMOR

Research has shown that optimistic people have better memories. People who believe that they can and will remember something are more likely to do so. In addition to a better memory, the benefits of optimism include a reduction in stress and depression, better overall health, increased self-esteem, and a longer life.

Closely aligned with optimism are humor and laughter, both of which reduce stress, increase relaxation, nurture optimism, reduce anxiety, promote health, and improve mood, all of which can have a positive and significant impact on memory. We have the ability to learn to become more optimistic and to introduce more humor into our lives, and we should all practice doing so to enhance memory.

NUTRITION

The benefits of sound nutrition have gained a lot of attention over the past few years. We have long known that good nutrition is good for the body, and increasingly we are finding that what we eat has a huge impact on memory as well. Three food groups are at the forefront of brain health—antioxidants, omega-3 fatty acids, and green, leafy vegetables. Antioxidants rid the body of free radicals, which can damage cells, and also help to improve blood flow to the brain. Dark-colored fruits and vegetables, such as berries, kale, spinach, and beets, are rich in antioxidants. Omega-3 fatty acids, found in certain types of fish and nuts, have been found to slow the rate of cognitive decline. And green, leafy vegetables, which are high in folic acid and B vitamins, are critical to keeping memory sharp.

Many other foods are good for the brain. What's good for the heart is also good for the brain. It's important to learn the recommended daily servings of food categories, because a well-rounded diet can help you to think more clearly and remember more efficiently.

SOCIALIZATION

Studies on socialization among adults and its effect on memory have shown that social participation and integration have profound effects on health and well-being throughout a person's lifetime. People with many social ties generally live longer and healthier lives, feel better about themselves, and have slower rates of memory decline. Socialization can indeed help people to maintain a healthy brain and memory.

We all need to make socialization an integral and continual part of our lives. We need to find ways to foster friendships, maintain family ties, make new friends, try new things, volunteer, and be passionate about life. There are many ways to do this, and it's important to explore a variety of these ways, not just those that are familiar to us.

Memory-Enhancement Course Review
FACILITATOR INSTRUCTIONS

1. ## WELCOME AND INTRODUCTION (5 MINUTES)

To do before class:

- Read and familiarize yourself with the Memory-Enhancement Course Overview.
- Write the following quotes on a board or flip chart.

> When I was younger, I could remember anything, whether it happened or not.
> (Mark Twain, author, humorist)

> Memory is what tells a man that his wife's birthday was yesterday.
> (Mario Rocco, entertainer)

- Prepare a certificate of completion for each participant.
- Familiarize yourself with and make appropriate copies of the warm-up activity, quiz, practice activities, and homework.
- Gather a variety of magazines as well as colored pens or pencils, scissors, glue or tape, and heavy 11×14 white paper.

Congratulate everybody on making it through the last 11 classes! Let the group know that the focus of this final class will be to review, integrate, and practice the information learned during the course. In a humorous way, discuss the significance of the quotes and their relationship to memory.

2. ## WARM-UP ACTIVITY (10 MINUTES)

A good way to begin a review of the 11 classes is to ask participants what they are doing or thinking of doing that is good for their brains that they learned from the classes. Pass out the worksheet *Good for the Brain* and give the group 5 minutes to complete it. Ask people to share their answers and also ask which beneficial things they have started doing since the course began.

3.   QUIZ (10 MINUTES)

Pass out the *Memory-Enhancement Review Quiz* and let participants know that the true or false statements are all based on information covered in the 11 classes. After allowing everyone 3 to 4 minutes to complete the quiz, review each answer, pausing for questions and comments.

4.   EDUCATION AND DISCUSSION (25 MINUTES)

Information from each class hopefully has built upon the ones before it and new techniques have been integrated into the memory of each participant. It is important to review each class in a concise manner with the group and to urge each participant to review each class more fully on his or her own.

Distribute and quickly review the handout *Memory-Enhancement Tips*, which includes recommendations from the 11 classes. Suggest to participants that they add any other tips that they think may be helpful and to post the list in a location where they can review it on a regular basis.

5.   PRACTICE ACTIVITIES (20 MINUTES)

Pass out the activity *A Collage of Memory Tips*. Place a variety of magazines, colored pens or pencils, glue or tape, and scissors on a table(s). Give participants 10 to 15 minutes to complete the activity. Suggest that if they are unable to complete the collage in time that they take some pictures home to work on it. Ask for one or two people to share their collage. Encourage participants to take their collage home and hang it up somewhere conspicuous where it can serve as an inspiration to continue working on ways to improve memory now that the course is coming to an end.

6.   REVIEW AND CLOSING CEREMONY (15 MINUTES)

Ask participants to name one or two tips or strategies that they learned in any of the classes that they have already used successfully. Discuss the importance of *practicing* all that they have learned in order to have the best memory possible. Depending on the group, you may want to suggest that they continue to have memory-enhancement get-togethers on their own time during which they can socialize and work on brain-stimulating activities such as games and puzzles.

Congratulate the group for making memory improvement an important part of their lives during the past 12 weeks (or however long the course has been going on). Thank them for their participation. Pass out certificates of completion to each person.

7.   HOMEWORK (5 MINUTES)

Pass out the homework sheets and explain what should be done for each. Remind participants of the importance of continuing to improve their brain fitness. One way to do this is to engage in mentally stimulating activities. Suggest that they set aside some time each day to do this. Encourage them to check for brain-stimulating activities in newspapers, online, in magazines, with friends, on the American Association for Retired Persons (AARP) Web site, in a library, and in a bookstore's puzzle section. Also, distribute to each participant a copy of the Resource List at the end of the book.

- *A–Z of Healthy Foods.* Using the A–Z format to list items in specific categories is both stimulating for the brain and fun to do. Once you have distributed the worksheet, brainstorm with the group other categories for which they could create a list of items using the A–Z format.

- *How Many Can You Name? Magazines, Magazines, Magazines!* After distributing the worksheet, ask participants for suggestions of other categories for which they would enjoy naming as many items as they can.

- *Old-Time Movie Favorites.* Reiterate to participants the importance of using their whole brain, being social, and having fun. One way to do these is to get together with friends or family and brainstorm a topic such as old movies, discussing as many aspects as possible.

Review of Classes 1–11
CLASS AGENDA

1. Welcome and Introduction
2. Warm-Up Activity
   - *Good for the Brain*
3. Quiz
   - *Memory-Enhancement Review Quiz*
4. Review of the Memory-Enhancement Course
   - *Memory-Enhancement Tips*
5. Practice Activities
   - *A Collage of Memory Tips*
6. Review and Closing Ceremony!
7. Homework
   - *A–Z of Healthy Foods*
   - *How Many Can You Name? Magazines, Magazines, Magazines!*
   - *Old-Time Movie Favorites*

Good for the Brain

Name 10 things that you currently do that are good for your brain.

1.

2.

3.

4.

5.

6.

7.

8.

9.

10.

Strengthen Your Mind Program: A Course for Memory Enhancement by Einberger & Sellick.

Memory-Enhancement Review Quiz

Answer the following statement with a *T* for *True* or an *F* for *False*.

_____ 1. Finding a new way to do something strengthens your mind more than doing it the same way as you have always done it.

_____ 2. Adults tend to laugh approximately the same amount of times each day as young children do.

_____ 3. People who walk for 2½ hours each week perform better on cognitive tests than those who don't.

_____ 4. All fruits and vegetables contain high levels of antioxidants.

_____ 5. If your primary learning style is visual, it is important that you see the person who is speaking.

_____ 6. Stress limits what and how much we remember.

_____ 7. As we grow older, we become less efficient at multitasking.

_____ 8. Most people use both sides of their brain—right and left—equally.

_____ 9. The sense of smell is the best at recalling memories.

_____ 10. Although optimism is a positive trait, being optimistic does not improve memory.

_____ 11. Socializing with others can slow mental decline.

_____ 12. Mnemonics are phrases that help you to remember lists or specific information.

_____ 13. Reading to yourself is more beneficial for your memory than reading aloud.

Strengthen Your Mind Program: A Course for Memory Enhancement by Einberger & Sellick.
© 2010 by Health Professions Press, Inc.

Memory-Enhancement Review Quiz ANSWER SHEET

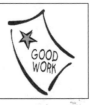

T   1.   Finding a new way to do something strengthens your mind more than doing it the same way as you have always done it.

F   2.   Adults tend to laugh approximately the same amount of times each day as young children do.

T   3.   People who walk for 2½ hours each week perform better on cognitive tests than those who don't.

F   4.   All fruits and vegetables contain high levels of antioxidants.

T   5.   If your primary learning style is visual, it is important that you see the person who is speaking.

T   6.   Stress limits what and how much we remember.

T   7.   As we grow older, we become less efficient at multitasking.

F   8.   Most people use both sides of their brain—right and left—equally.

T   9.   The sense of smell is the best at recalling memories.

F 10.   Although optimism is a positive trait, being optimistic does not improve memory.

T 11.   Socializing with others can slow mental decline.

T 12.   Mnemonics are phrases that help you to remember lists or specific information.

F 13.   Reading to yourself is more beneficial for your memory than reading aloud.

Strengthen Your Mind Program: A Course for Memory Enhancement by Einberger & Sellick.

Memory-Enhancement Tips

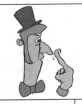

Pay attention. Concentrate on what you want to remember.

Take time to have fun.

Minimize distractions around you, such as excessive noise and movement.

Take care of your health.

Find ways to reduce stress in your life.

Keep your mind active by engaging in a variety of activities.

Socialize with others regularly.

Laugh often and freely.

Limit multitasking.

Listen to or play music.

Use your nondominant hand for routine activities, such as eating and writing. If you use the computer, try using the mouse with your nondominant hand.

Tune in to all of your senses.

Eat a heart-healthy diet.

Eat foods high in antioxidants.

Keep a positive attitude.

Keep your body active.

Use your dominant learning style, but don't neglect the use of the other two styles to augment your learning.

Use a variety of memory techniques to learn new information.

Enjoy life and continue to grow.

Strengthen Your Mind Program: A Course for Memory Enhancement by Einberger & Sellick.
© 2010 by Health Professions Press, Inc.

A Collage of Memory Tips

Create a collage of memory tips using colored pens or pencils, words, phrases, or pictures from magazines or newspapers. Include a variety of things that remind you of tips that you have learned in the 11 memory-enhancement classes, which are listed below. An example might be a picture of a fruit basket, which could remind you of eating foods rich in antioxidants.

Classes:

#1	Memory and Aging
#2	Learning Styles
#3	Mental Aerobics
#4	Exercise
#5	Strategies for Memory Improvement
#6	Brain Dominance
#7	The Five Senses
#8	Stress
#9	Optimism and Humor
#10	Nutrition
#11	Socialization

After you finish the collage, hang it somewhere where you will see it on a daily basis to remind yourself of ways that you can enhance your memory.

Strengthen Your Mind Program: A Course for Memory Enhancement by Einberger & Sellick.
© 2010 by Health Professions Press, Inc.

MEMORY ENHANCEMENT COURSE

THIS CERTIFIES THAT

has successfully completed the Strengthen Your Mind Course

GIVEN THIS _____ DAY OF _____, 20_____

_____
FACILITATOR

A–Z of Healthy Foods

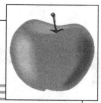

Using the alphabet as a way to remember things that you've learned is a great memory technique. Name at least one healthy food using each letter of the alphabet. For example, the letter *b* could be for *broccoli*. This is also a great activity for using all of your senses! Think of other topics for which you can create a list in this way (men's and women's names, famous people, things you might find at the circus, types of animals, colors).

A	N
B	O
C	P
D	Q
E	R
F	S
G	T
H	U
I	V
J	W
K	X
L	Y
M	Z

Strengthen Your Mind Program: A Course for Memory Enhancement by Einberger & Sellick.

How Many Can You Name?
Magazines, Magazines, Magazines!

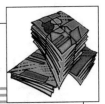

How many magazine titles can you list below? For more answers, go on-line or check the magazine section at the grocery store. Think of other categories you can use for naming as many items as you can (singers, trees, dairy products, stores, restaurants, flowers, cars). This is a great brain-fitness activity, and the sky is the limit!

1.

2.

3.

4.

5.

6.

7.

8.

9.

10.

11.

12.

13.

14.

15.

Strengthen Your Mind Program: A Course for Memory Enhancement by Einberger & Sellick.
© 2010 by Health Professions Press, Inc.

Old-Time Movie Favorites

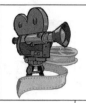

Talk about old movies with friends or family members.

Who were the stars?

Where and when did the movie take place?

What did the scenery look like?

How much did it cost to see the movie?

Did you buy snacks at the theater?

Were there special tastes or smells that you remember as you watched the movie?

Were the actors' voices clear?

Were there any special effects and, if so, which?

Strengthen Your Mind Program: A Course for Memory Enhancement by Einberger & Sellick.

Bibliography

Aamont, S., & Wang, S., (2008). *Welcome to Your Brain*. New York: Bloomsbury.

American Heritage College Dictionary. (2007). Boston: Houghton Mifflin Company.

Alzinfo.org. (2007). *More Coffee? It May Keep the Memory Sharp*. Retrieved March 2, 2009, from http://www.alzinfo.org/newsarticle/templates/newstemplate.asp?articleid=239&zoneid=10.

Anderson, J. (2009). *Can Exercising Your Brain Prevent Memory Loss?* Retrieved April 19, 2009, from http://www.eurekalert.org/pub_releases/2009-02/aaon-cey021009.php.

Basler, B. (2008). *Exercise May Slow the Ravages of Alzheimer's*. Retrieved March 22, 2009, from http://bulletin.aarp.org/yourhealth/diseases/articles/day_2__exercise_may.html.

Bauer, J. (2008). *Avoid Brain Drain with Memory Boosting Foods*. Retrieved March 3, 2009, from http://www.msnbc.msn.com/id/25572443/.

BBC News. (2009). *Knitting Can Delay Memory Loss*. Retrieved March 6, 2009, from http://news.bbc.co.uk/2/hi/health/7896441.stm.

Boerner, H. (n.d.). *50 Ways to Boost Your Noodle*. Retrieved January 12, 2009, from http://www.aarp.org/health/healthyliving/brain_health/articles/noodle_boosters.html.

Bragdon, A., & Monbleau, M. (1999). *Right Brain Teasers*. Bass River, MA: Allen D. Bragdon Publishers, Inc.

Crooks, V., Lubben J., Petitti, D., Little, D., & Chiu, V. (2008). *Social Network, Cognitive Function, and Dementia Incidence Among Elderly Women*. Retrieved April 5, 2009, from http://www.ajph.org/cgi/content/abstract/98/7/1221.

Daily Mail Reporter. (2008). *A Curry Could Help Boost Your Memory and Help Prevent Alzheimer's*. Retrieved April 23, 2009, from http://www.dailymail.co.uk/health/article-1043718/A-curry-help-boost-memory-prevent-Alzheimers.html.

Dew, J. (1996). *Are You a Right Brain or Left Brain Thinker?* Retrieved March 22, 2009, from http://bama.ua.edu/~st497/creative.html.

Diament, M. (2008). *Make New Friends, Get Involved: Socializing Is Good For Your Brain*. Retrieved March 22, 2009, from http://bulletin.aarp.org/yourhealth/diseases/articles/make_new_friends_get_involved_socializing_is_good_for_your_brain.html.

Einberger, K. (2008). *Sharpen Your Senses*. Verona, WI: Attainment Company, Inc.

Einberger, K., & Sellick, J. (2007). *Strengthen Your Mind: Activities for People with Early Memory Loss*. Baltimore: Health Professions Press.

Einberger, K., & Sellick, J. (2008). *Strengthen Your Mind: Activities for People Concerned About Early Memory Loss, Volume 2*. Baltimore: Health Professions Press.

Einstein, G. O., & McDaniel, M. A. (2003). *Memory Fitness: A Guide to Successful Aging*. New Haven, CT: Yale University Press.

Engleman, M. (2006). *Aerobics of the Mind.* Verona, WI: Attainment Company, Inc.

Ertel, K., Glymour, M., & Berkman, L. (2008). *Effects of Social Integration on Preserving Memory Function in a Nationally Representative U.S. Elderly Population.* Retrieved April 2, 2009, from http://www.ajph.org/cgi/content/abstract/98/7/1215.

Fielding, B. (1999). *The Memory Manual.* Clovis, CA: Quill Driver Books.

Finnemore, G. (2009). *Brain Fitness and Training Heads Towards Its Tipping Point.* Retrieved January 30, 2009, from http://www.sharpbrains.com/blog/2009/01/19/brain-fitness-training-heads-towards-its-tipping-point.

The Franklin Institute, Resources for Science Living. (n.d.). *Cortisol and Temporary Memory Loss Study.* Retrieved February 3, 2009, from http://www.fi.edu/learn/brain/stress.html.

Higbee, K. L. (1996). *Your Memory: How It Works and How to Improve It* (2nd ed.). New York: Marlowe and Company.

Jaffe-Gill, E., Rose, A., Kemp, G., & Barston, S. (2007). *Improving Your Memory: Tips and Techniques for Memory Enhancement.* Retrieved March 2, 2009, from http://www.helpguide.org/life/improving_memory.htm.

Janata, J. (2009). *Is There Really Good Stress and Bad Stress?* Retrieved February 3, 2009, from http://abcnews.go.com/print?id=4668140.

Kage, B. (2006). *Omega 3 Fatty Acids Help Prevent Dementia, US Study Suggests.* Retrieved July 3, 2009 from http://www.naturalnews.com/021100.html.

Latham, C. (2007). *Stress and Short-Term Memory.* Retrieved February 3, 2009, from http://www.sharpbrains.com/blog/2007/06/04/stress-and-short-term-memory/.

Lautenschlager et al. (2008). Effect of Physical Activity on Cognitive Function in Older Adults at Risk for Alzheimer's Disease. *Journal of the American Medical Association, 300* (9), 1027–1037.

Lavelle, P. (2003). *Music Improves Language and Memory.* Retrieved April 20, 2009, from http://www.abc.net.au/science/articles/2003/07/29/911523.htm.

Martinuzzi, B. (2006). *Optimism: The Hidden Asset.* Retrieved March 8, 2009, from http://www.mindtools.com/pages/article/newLDR_72.htm.

McKeever, K. (2009). Simple Exercise Keeps Brain at Top of Its Game. Retrieved March 13, 2009, from http://www.medicinenet.com/script/main/art.asp?articlekey=95913.

McPherson, F. (2005). *Does Physical Exercise Improve Cognitive Function?* Retrieved March 13, 2009, from http://www.memory-key.com/strategies/exercise.

Mountain State Centers for Independent Living. *Understanding and Dealing with Stress.* Retrieved February 2, 2009, from http://www.mtstcil.org/skills/stress-definition-1.html.

Nelson, A. P. (2005). *The Harvard Medical School Guide to Achieving Optimal Memory.* Boston: McGraw-Hill.

Nussbaum, P. (2003). *Brain Health and Wellness.* Tarentum: PA: Word Association Publishers.

O'Brien, D. (2000). *Learn to Remember: Practical Techniques and Exercises to Improve Your Memory.* San Francisco: Chronicle Books.

O'Brien, J. (2008). *Age-Related Memory Loss Tied to Slip in Filtering Information Quickly.* Retrieved September 3, 2008, from http://www.ucsfhealth.org/adult/health_library/news/2008/09/119948.html.

O'Donnell, L. (1999). *Music and the Brain.* Retrieved April 20, 2009, from http://www.cerebromente.org.br/n15/mente/musica.html.

Perrig-Chiello, P., Perrig, W. J., Ehrsam, R., Staeheljn, H. B., & Krings, F. (1998). The Effects of Resistance Training on Well-being and Memory in Elderly Volunteers. *Age and Ageing, 27,* 469–475.

Pines, M. (2008). *The Mystery of Smell: The Vivid World of Odors.* Retrieved March 20, 2009, from http://hhmi.org/senses/d110.html.

Piper, W. (1976). *The Little Engine that Could.* New York: Golden Press.

Proust, M. (2006). *Remembrance of Things Past, Volume One.* Hertfordshire, U.K.: Wordsworth Edition, Ltd.

Ritchie, K. et al. (2007). The Neuroprotective Effects of Caffeine: A Prospective Population Study. *Neurology, 69,* 536–545.

Rush University Medical Center. (2006). *Social Networks Protect Against Alzheimer's.* Retrieved June 17, 2009, from http://www.sciencedaily.com–/releases/2006/04/060421234704.htm.

SeniorJournal.com. (2004). *People with Early Alzheimer's Can Still Learn, Study Says.* Retrieved April 3, 2009, from http://seniorjournal.com/NEWS/Alzheimers/4-07-10StillLearn.htm.

The Thinking Business. (n.d.). *The Herman Brain Dominance Instrument.* Retrieved March 7, 2009, from http://www.thethinkingbusiness.co.uk/hbdi.html.

University of California–Irvine. (2008). *Short-term Stress Can Affect Learning and Memory.* Retrieved February 3, 2009, from http://www.sciencedaily.com/releases/2008/03/080311182434.htm.

Vaillant, G. E. (2002). *Aging Well: Surprising Guideposts to a Happier Life.* New York: Little Brown.

Visual, Auditory, and Kinesthetic Survey. Retrieved June 26, 2009, from http://www.vark-learn.com/english/page.asp?p=questionnaire.

Resource List

BOOKS

Aerobics of the Mind Cards: 100 Exercises for a Healthy Brain, by Marge Engleman. Published by Attainment Company (www.attainmentcompany.com).

Aging Well: Surprising Guideposts to a Happier Life from the Landmark Harvard Study of Adult Development, by George Vaillant. Published by Little, Brown and Company.

Brain Health and Wellness, by Dr. Paul Nussbaum. Published by Word Association Publishers.

The Harvard Medical Guide to Achieving Optimal Memory, by Aaron Nelson. Published by Harvard College.

Learn to Remember: Practical Techniques and Exercises to Improve Your Memory, by Dominic O'Brien. Published by Chronicle Books.

Managing Your Memory: Practical Solutions for Forgetting, by Bill Beckwith. Published by Memory Management (www.memorymanagement.info).

The Memory Manual: Ten Simple Things You Can Do to Improve Your Memory after 50, by Betty Fielding. Published by Quill Driver Books (www.quilldriverbooks.com).

Mind Your Mind: A Whole Brain Workout for Older Adults, by Beatrice Seagull. Published by Attainment Company (www.attainmentcompany.com).

Right Brain Teasers, by Allen D. Bragdon and Marcia J. Monbleau. Published by Allen D. Bragdon Publishers, Inc.

Right Brain Teasers: A Photo Quiz for the Mind's Eye, by Allen D. Bragdon and Marcia J. Monbleau. Published by Brainwaves Books (www.brainwaves.com).

Sharpen Your Senses Activity Cards, by Kristin Einberger. Published by the Attainment Company (www.attainmentcompany.com).

Strengthen Your Mind: Activities for People Concerned About Early Memory Loss, Volume 2, by Kristin Einberger and Janelle Sellick. Published by Health Professions Press (www.healthpropress.com).

Strengthen Your Mind: Activities for People With Early Memory Loss, Volume 1, by Kristin Einberger and Janelle Sellick. Published by Health Professions Press (www.healthpropress.com).

Welcome to Your Brain: Why You Lose Your Car Keys but Never Forget to Drive and Other Puzzles of Everyday Life, by Sam Wang and Sandra Aamodt. Published by Bloomsbury Publishing.

Your Memory: How It Works and How to Improve It, by Kenneth Higbee. Published by Marlowe and Company.

WEB SITES

Ageless Learner (www.agelesslearner.com). Offers new approaches to learning.

American Association of Retired Persons (www.aarp.org). Information about general health, wellness, and memory on this site for persons age 50 and older.

A Learning Styles Survey for College (written by Catherine Jester) (http://www.meta math.com/multiple/multiple_choice_questions.html). A questionnaire that assesses which senses a person uses most effectively to take in information. Suggestions on how to use perceptual abilities are provided.

Lumosity (www.lumosity.com). A great subscription site. Offers a brain-training program that consists of engaging brain games and exercises.

Memory Improvement (www.memory-improvement-tips.com). Provides a wide variety of tips for memory improvement.

The Memory Key (www.memory-key.com). Offers many articles, tips, and ideas for memory improvement.

Mind Tools (www.mindtools.com). Designed for improving careers, although it is also filled with valuable information on general life enhancement.

People Quiz (www.peoplequiz.com). A variety of trivia.

Sharp Brains (www.sharpbrain.com). A research-based Web site focused on brain fitness and cognitive health.

Vark, A Guide to Learning Styles (http://www.vark-learn.com/english/page.asp?p= questionnaire). A questionnaire that assesses a person's preferred learning style(s).